HOLISTIC APPROACH

TO

RESTORATIVE SLEEP

Author: Bikramjit Konwar

This book has been dedicated to all without whom I will never be able to write this book and who supported me in this process.

Disclaimer:

The Information contained in this book is not designed to substitute or take place or provide any form of medical or professional advice or diagnose, treat, cure and prevent any disease. Information in this book has been provided solely for informational, educational, and entertainment purposes.

Everyone can have different health status, and the same foods of lifestyle strategies work well for one may not have the same result for others. You should not apply any of the Information, whether foods, lifestyle strategies, or any other information mentioned in this book before consultation with your doctor or healthcare professionals with knowledge on the subject.

Under no circumstances will any legal responsibility or blame be held against the author/publisher/copyrighter for any reparation, damages, injury, monetary loss, or any undesirable consequences resulting from the application of any information provided by this book either directly or indirectly.

By purchasing, downloading, and/or reading this book, you agree that you have read this statement and accept all the risks of using the Information presented inside this book.

ABOUT THE AUTHOR:

The author, Bikramjit Konwar, was born in 1976. He had lost health due to the poor lifestyle and food habits. After years of struggling, he recovered health by adopting food and lifestyle strategies. Later the author earned a Diploma in Nutrition and also Naturopath. He spent several years in the advanced study of health and well-being and super passionate about learning. Food is the one most crucial thing for health- no one is arguing that. But other lifestyle factors like behavior, stress handling, sleep, physical activeness, and other well-being measures are no less crucial towards a healthy life. It is vital what tools and strategies we have, what fits our lives, and how we can implement them to achieve sustainable health and happiness. The author likes to help people and share the knowledge he gained and lacking that he had suffered severely in the past. The author has a specific interest in Longevity, Health-span, Happiness, Nature, and Environment.

Courses the author has completed further presently, and the learning process is never going to be an end.

- Weight Management: Beyond Balancing Calories created by Professor Sharon Horesh Bergquist authorized by Emory University
- The Science of Well-Being created by Cognitive Scientist and Professor Laurie Santos authorized by Yale University
- Autophagy: Research Behind the 2016 Nobel Prize in Physiology or Medicine provided by Nobel Prize winner Prof. Yoshinori Ohsumi and Research Team offered by University of Tokyo Institute of Technology

TABLE OF CONTENTS:

A call from a Friend

Recently, I had a call from one of my fitness enthusiasts friends. He has enough will power and spends hours in the gym. Even so, he was struggling to lose body fat and abnormal blood lipids. After a few discussions about food habits and lifestyle, I asked him about his sleep. I was shocked when he told me he was doing his job and other daily activities at his sleep expense. Simultaneously, he has a strong mentality and enough willpower and doing all this because of his strong will power. I have recently heard from another friend who was struggling to lose weight. She was a regular user of gadgets to the late-night at the expense of sleep. But they are not alone who are doing in such ways.

Many of us are making a similar approach is at the expense of sleep and ending with weight gain and killing our health. That develops several chronic diseases particularly metabolic diseases. We keep our daily sleep to fulfil at the weakened. But that strategy doesn't work and results in killing health. Scientists always warn about this strategy.

Healthy eating is one most important thing for a healthy and joyful life. No one is arguing that. You may or may not know what healthy eating is. But even you know what healthy eating is, it is hard to eat healthy if you are sleep deprived, depressed, and life is full of stress and dissatisfaction. Remember, the human body has the one most complex mechanism ever built on this planet-that no one has clearly understood this. A human body never works isolated or part by part; all are connected by biochemical messengers like neurotransmitters. For sustainable health, your foods need to be healthful, tasteful, and satisfying- which is a different story. You can't run long with boring foods. I am coming on these with a separate book.

At this beginning of this book, we will explore how bad things can happen in someone's health who does not have enough sleep. How can someone gain extra weight with an experience of impaired sleep habits?

Why do you need good sleep?

According to sleep research scientist Teresa Arora, Ph.D., *"Sleep doesn't waste time; it's good for the waistline."* (1)

Sleep and health are inextricably connected

A night of good sleep is restorative. A night of uninterrupted sleep leaves your body and mind rejuvenated for the next day. Sleep has important roles in the metabolism of foods you eat, your emotional and cognitive-behavioral regulation. Today, insufficient sleep has become a growing global problem. Unfortunately, in the last 40 years alone, the average sleep duration has decreased by two hours. However, this depends not only on a single factor. Sleep deprivation can be attributed to multiple factors, such as workload, lifestyle, food intake, social activities, and technology. (2)

You need good sleep for muscle repair, memory consolidation, and the release of hormones that regulate your growth and appetite. A short sleep impairs these processes. You wake up less prepared to concentrate, make decisions, or engage fully in school or work, and other social activities-National Sleep Foundation explained. (3)

Brain health, Clears brain toxins

Sleep is extremely important to brain health. Our memory, cognitive, and decision-making ability may go down with sleep deprivation. And many of our day-to-day lifestyle decision can go wrong with less sleep.

In a study, sleep had increased clearance of toxins like beta-amyloid, which can contribute to Alzheimer's disease in mice. (4) Other studies also found the link between sleep deprivation and the process of loss and functions of neurons and cognitive impairment. (5)

In a recent study, investigators at Harvard-affiliated Brigham and Women's Hospital explored the connection between sleep disturbances and deficiencies among older adults and the risk of dementia and death. They found the risk of dementia was two-fold higher among participants who were sleeping fewer than five hours of sleep per night compared to those who were sleeping seven to eight hours of sleep per night. The researchers also found associations between sleep disturbances and sleep deficiency with the overall risk of death. (6)

Your body needs to clear toxins, daily metabolic wastes from your brain. The restorative function of sleep cleans toxins, metabolic waste products from the brain. To find out how sleep clears toxins from the brain, researchers from Boston University conducted a study. During a phase of sleep, they found neurons in the brain start to synchronize, and large oscillations of fluid inflow to the brain appeared during sleep. That draws cerebrospinal fluid into and out of the brain. Cerebrospinal fluid clears metabolic waste products from the brain and protects the brain tissue from injury. (7)

Does sleep can be replaced by rest?

A recent study evidenced sleep is more than rest for plasticity in the human cortex. Brain plasticity or neuroplasticity is the capacity of our neurons and neural networks in the brain to change their connections and behavior in response to new information, sensual inputs, development, damage, or dysfunction. We need it for the right answer to our external circumstances.

In this study, researchers found, sleep-specific brain activity is superior to an equal period of rest for improved brain performance and can't be replaced. The state of the brain is unique during sleep and is required to restore wake-associated deterioration. (8)

CHAPTER 2

Sleep deprivation, Food Craving, weight gain, and many health disorders

We have talked, with sleep deprivation, your body and brain don't function properly, unknowingly you are not in your control, and many things can go wrong. Numerous studies have reported the negative impact of inadequate sleep on brain structure, activation as well as physiology. (1)

Sleep deprivation or inadequate sleep impairs both mental health as well as physical health and increases stress levels. (2, 3)

But the problems don't end here.

You lose cognitive function, control, and your brain will search for comfort, pleasures from the outside world. Many of your decisions, including eating behavior, choice of foods can go wrong, and you will not be in the driving seat of your eating behavior. People with less sleep tend to eat morehigh-glycemic and unhealthy comfort foods, particularly desserts/sweets/snacks, to please the brain. In today's world, such foods' consumption is the primary reason to kill our health and gain weight.

Low level of satisfaction hormone and high level of the hunger hormone and increased consumption of unhealthy foods

Again this is not the whole story. With sleep deprivation, the level of two important hormones, leptin and ghrelin, become altered. Hormone leptin gives you satiety from foods and tells your brain to stop eating. And the hunger hormone ghrelin tells you to eat more. The level of ghrelin spikes, while the level of leptin falls. (4)

Researchers at the University of Chicago had conducted a study on peoples who slept only four hours a night for two nights. They found with sleep deprivation, the participant's leptin level decreased by 18 percent, ghrelin level increased by 28 percent, hunger level increased by 24 percent with a surge in desire for calorie-dense, high-carbohydrate processed snacks and comfort foods. (5)

In another study, researchers from several universities assessed the effect of five hours in bed per night for four nights and found sleep restriction decreased the participants' satiety. (6)

That could be another reason to eat more, as you don't feel so full after eating.

With decreased satiety, other studies also found that short sleepers had higher calorie intakes. But that is not the end; they notably consumed more from unhealthy comfort foods like sugar-sweetened beverages, desserts, sweets, and snacks than normal sleepers do. Several studies reported similar results. (7, 8, 9, 10)

Cognitive function, decision making, brain reward

You may feel how hard it is to eat healthily when your brain is exhausted and looking for comfort, even when you know about the importance of healthy eating.

Another reason: unhealthy comfort foods or food-like substances stimulate a hormone called dopamine that provides brain reward, a pleasure to the brain.

This inclination to unhealthy comfort foods is because of pleasure in the brain, impaired cognitive decision making of your brain. But that doesn't do any good to your health. Instead, those minutes of pleasure bombard your health. Chronic sleep deprivation may change eating behavior, and that can lead to a greater propensity to overeat. Several scientific studies have supported that. In adolescents, sleep restriction aggravates mood and emotion regulation. And high glycemic index foods like sweets/desserts were more appealing to adolescents after sleep restriction. Several studies observed similar results. (11, 12, 13, 14, 15, 16)

Low insulin sensitivity, high blood sugar, & Diabetes

Moreover, sleep deprivation results in impaired carbohydrate metabolism, which means your body can't handle the carbohydrates you eat in the right way. Getting poor sleep has been linked to high blood sugar levels in people with diabetes and prediabetes. Sleep loss affects insulin, the stress hormone cortisol, and oxidative stress. (17)

An increased level of oxidative stress means our body is unable to neutralize harmful highly reactive free radicals effectively. That results in tissue damage leading to chronic diseases.

- Several clinical studies found, sleep deprivation impairs insulin sensitivity and results in an insulin-resistant state (18, 19, 20)
- In another clinical study, researchers from University of California and Touro University measured sleep restriction decreased whole-body insulin resistance by 25% compared to normal (21)
- And even one night's sleep deprivation can impair fasting insulin sensitivity in healthy men (22, 23)

When your cells have low insulin sensitivity or a state of insulin resistance, your blood sugar level becomes high and opens the door to diabetes.

Studies have also found that later or irregular sleeping schedules are correlated with higher blood sugar, even in non-diabetic people. (17, 24, 25)

In another clinical study, researchers from Diabetes and Obesity Research Institute, Los Angeles, University of Chicago, and more found sleep restriction in healthy men results in an increased level of free fatty acids. They also concluded that this might partly contribute to insulin resistance and the elevated diabetes risk associated with sleep loss. (26) Longtime sleep deprivation can increase the risk of obesity, type 2 diabetes. (27, 28)

In summary, many studies found that loss of sleep can lead to adverse health effects, including increased daytime sleepiness, impaired mood, cognitive function and daytime performance, increased insulin resistance, change of eating behavior with eating a high amount of comfort foods. These increase inflammation inside the body and cause impaired blood sugar regulation. (29, 30, 31, 32)

Immune Function

We all know how important the immune system is for our health, wound healing, and protection against chronic diseases and life-threatening diseases.   With growing research, it is now increasingly clear that sleep and immune function are closely interrelated.   For example, researchers found sound sleep improves T cells, a type of vital immune cells. (33)

A recent study found sleep hormone melatonin secretion in the lung acts as a barrier against the COVID-19 virus. The researchers found melatonin encodes proteins used for defence in the nose, lungs to prevent the virus entry so that the virus remains in the respiratory tract for few days. That activates the immune system and triggers the production of antibodies against the virus. (34)That may explain why some people are not infected or don't show symptoms even diagnosed as carriers of the virus.

Research also suggests that sleep strengthens immune memory against harmful antigens. While proper sleep strengthens the immune system's effectiveness and well functioning, lack of sleep impairs these processes. (35)

Studies show that sleep loss can affect different parts of the immune system, leading to the development of a wide variety of disorders. For example, sleep reduces the activity of natural killer cells of our immune system. Reduced functioning of Natural Killer cells was associated with a 1.6 times higher risk of dying with cancer (all sites) in an 11-year follow-up study. Similarly, restricting sleep to 4 hours for one night led to the generation of inflammatory cytokines, which play an important role in developing cardiovascular and metabolic disorders. (35, 36)

Reduced lifespan, and many chronic diseases

An increased level of inflammation and impaired blood sugar regulation contribute to the development of many other chronic diseases and reduces lifespan. Although other drivers exist, these are the primary drivers of many current chronic health issues. Many people use a strategy to complete their demanding work with less sleep on weekdays and try to recover it later. And some keep it to recover at the weekend. Scientists warn that weekend recovery sleep may not sufficiently reverse all the sleep loss effects during the workweek. (29, 37, 38)

The uncontrolled consumption of comfort foods with refined sugar and processed carbohydrates, especially from sugar-sweetened foods, beverages, and processed foods, has enough power to kill your health. These toxic foods or food like substances are the primary reason for the development of numerous chronic health disorders. If you seek health, energetic movement, longevity, and then lose the extra weight by cutting out those foods, sleep is a top priority.

Other health issues with sleep disorders

Many health authorities, scientists warn that insufficient sleep can lead to serious health problems. Sleep disorders and chronic sleep loss can put you at risk for (39, 40, 41, 42)

- Weight gain and obesity
- High blood pressure
- Diabetes

- Heart disease and stroke
- Impaired immunity
- Depression
- Cognitive decline
- Alzheimer's disease and more

It is also crucial to understand that you are hungry or going to eat because you feel uncomfortable due to your sleep deprivation. That is what your brain is seeking, comfort foods for pleasure and an instant source of energy with sleep deprivation. According to the Mayo Clinic, in general, an adult needs 7-9 hour' uninterrupted night-time sleep in a day. The National Sleep Foundation also has a similar view. (43, 44)You may also find some people telling you that they do yoga or meditation; they need only a few hours of sleep. Here we are not talking about that.

So, next, what we are going explore in this book are

- Circadian Rhythm responds to the sleep-wake cycle, the sleep hormone, the best time to go to bed, food metabolism, and the body's direction while sleeping.
- Foods, nutrients that promote better sleep along
- Macronutrients participation in sleep, i.e., type of carbohydrates, fats, and proteins and their roles
- Evening foods & beverages, nutrients that hurt sleep, and what are the alternate options we have
- What habit, activities, things can hurt your sleep, prevent the release of sleep hormone?
- Strategies to go to sleep and calm your racing mind before bed, creating a better bedroom environment.
- Stress is an integral part of everyone's life. But uncontrollable stress can hurt our sleep at night apart from other health and lifestyle factors. Lesser-known strategies needed to handle stress in day to day life.
- We will talk about goal setting, happiness, what is important in life, and wellbeing science and lifestyle strategies.

- Other sides of exercises (lesser-known sides, we will not talk about muscle building or strength or cardio), what type, how much, and when? And how to incorporate exercises in a busy daily life.

We will go step by step and find the hidden facts in the above subjects. I am not good at writing. So, forgive me for any mistakes in my writings.

CHAPTER 3

What is the best time for sleep -Circadian Rhythm

In 2017, the Nobel Prize in Physiology or Medicine was awarded to Jeffrey C. Hall, Michael Rosbash, and Michael W. Young "for their discoveries of molecular mechanisms controlling the circadian rhythm" in fruit flies. (1)

Circadian rhythms influence our sleep-wake cycles, hormone release, eating habits and digestion, body temperature, and other critical bodily functions. Biological clocks that run fast or slow can result in disrupted or abnormal circadian rhythms. Irregular rhythms have been linked to various chronic health conditions, such as sleep disorders, obesity, diabetes, depression, bipolar disorder, and seasonal affective disorder. Although natural factors within the body produce circadian rhythms, signals from the external environment can affect them. The primary cue influencing circadian rhythms is daylight. This light can turn on or turn off genes that control the molecular structure of biological clocks. Changing the light-dark cycles can speed up, slow down, or reset biological clocks as well as circadian rhythms. (2)

And probably due to that reason, shift workers showed changes in eating behavior with the consumption of more unhealthy comfort foods and soft drinks seeking pleasure. (3,4)

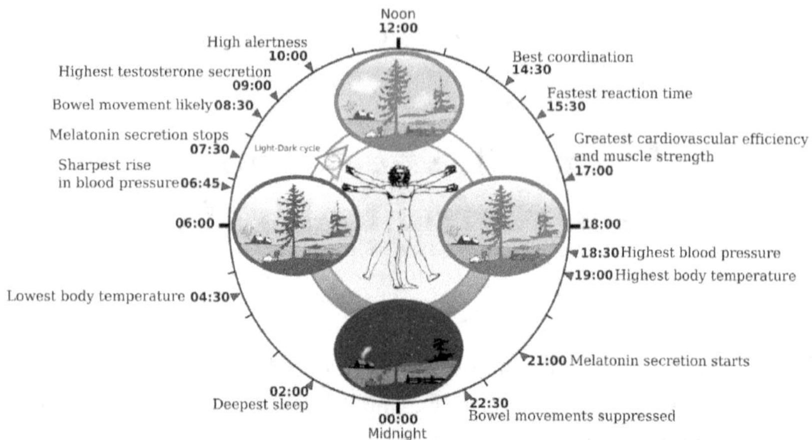

Source: Inkscape by YassineMrabet. Informations were provided from "The Body Clock Guide to Better Health" by Michael Smolensky and Lynne Lamberg; Henry Holt and Company, Publishers (2000)
https://en.wikipedia.org/wiki/Circadian_rhythm

Your brain produces the hormone melatonin in response to darkness. Melatonin is the hormone that tells you to go to bed. If you keep your light on at night during sleep, it can prevent melatonin production. If you see the biological circadian clock in humans, melatonin secretion starts at 9 pm, and accordingly, after some time, bowel movement is suppressed, and at 2 am, the deepest sleep occurs. (1)Therefore, your best time to sleep is between 9 pm to 6.30 am in general. Within this period, your sleep will be better and deeper, and there is less light to interfere with Circadian rhythms.

However, it is known that the beginning of the biological night for melatonin onset may differ from person to person, depending on their circadian timing or chronotype. Your chronotype shows you when to sleep based on the biological night of your internal clock. For example, people with early chronotypes present early melatonin onsets (around 7 pm), while late chronotypes have late melatonin onsets (around 1 am). (6) However, an individual may fall somewhere in between, who may not be an early chronotype or late chronotype.

Depending on your circadian typology or chronotype, your alertness may vary in the morning and evening. Knowing your chronotype helps to plan your activities efficiently based on your internal clock.

Center for Environmental Therapeutics (https://cet.org/) offered a Morningness-Eveningness Questionnaire to check the chronotype of an individual. You can check your chronotype by answering the questionnaire with the following two links:

Automated Morningness-Eveningness Questionnaire (AutoMEQ)-Center for Environmental Therapeutics

Morningness -Eveningness Questionnaire- Automated https://www.cet-surveys.com/index.php?sid=61524&newtest=Y

I am not endorsed or affiliated with Center for Environmental Therapeutics. Alternatively, you can go to my site, and there you will find the link for the automated version and also a downloadable pdf version. https://www.holistichealthnlife.com/meal-time-metabolic-health-chronotype/

It is also known that late chronotypes tend to eat late at night and have a higher risk of metabolic disturbances related to unhealthy lifestyle factors in food selection, physical activity, and sleep. Indeed, evening chronotypes show stress mostly when they get home late and have difficulties controlling the amount of food eaten. They present a higher tendency to consume unhealthy foods and alcoholic beverages. One extreme example of unhealthy eating behavior is also shift workers with an increased risk of obesity. (5)

While a morning chronotype type prefers to go to early bed and rise early, evening types desire a later bedtime and rise time. Researchers reported that melatonin impairs glucose tolerance. That means if you have late-night dinner with more carbohydrates, your glucose tolerance goes downside and this situation increases the probability of glucose-related metabolic disorders. (5)Frequent higher calorie consumption at late night increases the probability of metabolic dysfunction and being obese. (6)

Whatever your chronotype is, listen to the response of your own body; it is wiser to go to sleep when you feel tired and sleepy and wake up when you've had enough rest

The National Sleep Foundation suggests that the best time to fall asleep is somewhere between 8 pm and 12 am. (7)

Head Direction during Sleep

Although it needs more research, there may be reasons to consider the direction of sleep. We know that we have iron particles in our blood circulation that can respond to the magnetic field.

And the Earth creates its magnetic field from the electric currents generated in the liquid iron-nickel core. The Magnetic North Pole is where the Earth's magnetic field points vertically downward.

However, the magnetic North and South Pole are not aligned with the Geographic North and South Pole. There are some deviations in angles between magnetic and geographic poles. It is better directed by the compass. (8, 9)

The Earth's magnetic field (EMF) is the one that can influence a human's life, along with animals and birds.

In eastern practice, Vastu Shastra suggests laying down with your head pointed southward so that the magnetic field can interact optimally. (10)

A paper published in the Acta Medica International, a publication of Teerthanker Mahaveer University, reported- a study showed that those who were instructed to sleep with head in south direction for 12 weeks had the lowest systolic blood pressure, diastolic blood pressure, heart rate, and low level of stress. (11)

Although we need more research in this field, keeping the head to the north while sleeping may not be a good idea. And if you feel better by altering the direction, it may be worth try.

CHAPTER 4

Nutrients and Foods that promote better sleep

Like many other health issues, foods always take part in our sleep. When some foods, nutrients promote better sleep, and some other foods oppose it. In this chapter, we will find out what foods and nutrients can help us for better sleep. And in the next section, we will find what foods can hurt our sleep.

Melatonin rich foods

We already learned that when our body secretes the hormone melatonin, it signals to us that it's time to go to bed. Clinical studies found that when someone eats melatonin foods at night, it helps induce sleep, improve sleep quality, morning alertness, etc. Studies also reported that melatonin consumption two hours before bed improves sleep induction and quality in cancer patients with sleep insomnia. (1, 2, 3)

Tart cherries have a high dietary melatonin concentration.

In two different clinical studies, adult people with sleep difficulties who drank 8 ounces or 237 ml of tart cherry juice in the morning and one to two hours before bedtime for two weeks reported sleeping longer. They had better sleep quality in comparison to when they did not drink the juice. (4, 5) Other clinical studies have also found similar results. (6, 7)

Similarly, kiwi fruit can also promote sleep.

In a four-week study, people who ate two kiwifruits one hour before bedtime reported improvement in total sleep time and sleep efficiency. Moreover, the time required to fall asleep and waking time after sleep decreased. (8)

Kiwi fruit is beneficial for sleep because it contains a sleep-promoting component, as well as relaxing and protecting components, such as melatonin, magnesium, antioxidants, folate, and more. (9)

Some other foods that have a higher source of naturally occurring melatonin include: (10)

Animal products (fish, egg, meat, milk)

Fruits and vegetables (tart cherries, grapes, strawberries, tomato, mushroom, pepper)

Grains (black rice, red rice, rice, rolled oats)

Nuts and seeds contain varying amounts of melatonin.

However, you should also know that melatonin concentration in foods may vary, depending upon factors like temperature, the time exposed to sunlight, the ripening process, agrochemical treatment, etc.

Amino acid Tryptophan

Researchers found depletion of precursors of feel good and wellbeing neurotransmitter serotonin increased depressive moods. Tryptophan is an amino acid that is a building block of protein. You can't directly get serotonin from food, but you can have dietary amino acid tryptophan that's converted to serotonin. (1) Which is further converted to the sleep hormone melatonin. (2)

You may have heard that drinking milk at night helps to sleep better. This is because dairy foods contain tryptophan. (3)Moreover, studies found that people experiencing depression may have a low level of tryptophan, (4)

The precursor to melatonin is serotonin. (5) Several studies have shown that tryptophan-rich foods improve sleep by increasing melatonin. One study found the combination of tryptophan-rich breakfast and exposure to bright light during the daytime could promote melatonin secretion at night and better sleep. (6, 7, 8)

Foods that help to get tryptophan include poultry, shrimp, egg (with yolk), salmon, crab, spirulina, nuts, seeds, cheese, spinach, cereal grains, vegetables, and some more. (9)

It has been estimated that a typical diet provides about 1 gram per day. The daily nutritional requirement for tryptophan is modest (5 mg/kg). However, many adults choose to consume much more, up to 4-5 g/d (60-70 mg/kg), typically to improve mood or sleep. (10) Taking excess is not preferable as we have other ways to improve sleep.

Tryptophan works with vitamin B6, B3 or niacin, and magnesium to synthesize serotonin. Complex carbohydrates help make tryptophan more available in the brain, but high protein with tryptophan has the opposite effect. (1) As carbohydrates make tryptophan more available to the brain, that explains why carbohydrate-heavy meals can make you drowsy. (11) On the other hand, excess protein has the opposite effect. (1) That is probably due to similar structural proteins that may compete for each other for their position.

Also, clubbing protein with carbohydrates stimulates insulin to a higher level. (12, 13) Lesser use of insulin or the use of insulin within the specified limit is a strategy for longevity. Higher use of insulin makes disease-prone. That's why the combination of high carbohydrates and protein is also detrimental.

Therefore you need to balance this, not too much.

A combination of a moderate amount of protein foods containing tryptophan and complex carbohydrates may make it easier. (11)

Tryptophan helps you to fall asleep, but that doesn't mean that you need to overeat tryptophan. More is not always better, and moderation is the key.

Magnesium

The mineral magnesium is a great relaxer. In several ways, magnesium helps us to relax our bodies and tissues. In animal studies, researchers found that melatonin-rich foods and minerals like magnesium can regulate melatonin production. (1, 2) In a human clinical study, magnesium supplementation was shown to increase melatonin concentration in older adults. (3)

Another clinical study showed older people taking magnesium at a dose of 500mg per day had fallen asleep faster with improved sleep quality and reduced insomnia symptoms. (4) Other clinical studies also found improvement in sleep, quality of life, and a decrease in the stress hormone cortisol. (5, 6) A diet with sufficient magnesium and low aluminum is associated with deeper, less interrupted sleep. (7)

The daily dose for magnesium

Recommended Dietary Allowances (RDAs) for Magnesium: (8)

Age	Male	Female	Pregnancy	Lactation
Birth to 6 months	30 mg*	30 mg*		
7–12 months	75 mg*	75 mg*		
1–3 years	80 mg	80 mg		
4–8 years	130 mg	130 mg		
9–13 years	240 mg	240 mg		
14–18 years	410 mg	360 mg	400 mg	360 mg
19–30 years	400 mg	310 mg	350 mg	310 mg
31–50 years	420 mg	320 mg	360 mg	320 mg
51+ years	420 mg	320 mg		

Food Sources of Magnesium

Some food sources of magnesium: (8)

Food	Milligrams (mg) per serving	Percent DV*
Almonds, dry roasted, 1 ounce	80	20
Spinach, boiled, ½ cup	78	20
Cashews, dry roasted, 1 ounce	74	19
Peanuts, oil roasted, ¼ cup	63	16
Cereal, shredded wheat, 2 large biscuits	61	15
Soymilk, plain or vanilla, 1 cup	61	15
Black beans, cooked, ½ cup	60	15
Edamame, shelled, cooked, ½ cup	50	13
Peanut butter, smooth, 2 tablespoons	49	12
Avocado, cubed, 1 cup	44	11
Potato, baked with skin, 3.5 ounces	43	11
Rice, brown, cooked, ½ cup	42	11
Yogurt, plain, low fat, 8 ounces	42	11
Oatmeal, instant, 1 packet	36	9
Kidney beans, canned, ½ cup	35	9
Banana, 1 medium	32	8
Salmon, Atlantic, farmed, cooked, 3 ounces	26	7
Milk, 1 cup	24–27	6–7
Halibut, cooked, 3 ounces	24	6

Food	Milligrams (mg) per serving	Percent DV*
Raisins, ½ cup	23	6
Chicken breast, roasted, 3 ounces	22	6
Beef, ground, 90% lean, pan-broiled, 3 ounces	20	5
Broccoli, chopped and cooked, ½ cup	12	3
Rice, white, cooked, ½ cup	10	3
Apple, 1 medium	9	2
Carrot, raw, 1 medium	7	2

You can get magnesium from various food sources, such as leafy greens, nuts, legumes, seeds, and more. You may also find magnesium in some fortified foods. Foods like nuts, seeds, legumes, etc. contain anti-nutrients that interfere with the nutrients' absorption—the best way to have such foods is to soak them in water or sprouted. Unsweetened almond milk at night may also help you to relax and have a better sleep. Remember, if you are taking supplements and foods both, the combined effect may exceed the daily value.

B vitamins

Earlier, we said that tryptophan works with vitamin B6, niacin, or B3. A small clinical crossover study showed that vitamin B-12 affects plasma melatonin concentrations and contributes to the light-dark cycle's entrainment. (1)

Another study found an association of vitamin B-12 with improvements in sleep quality and alertness. (2,3) Typically, the B vitamin group works together. An example is vitamin B9 or folate works together with

Vitamin B12 to support some of the most fundamental cell division processes and replication processes. (4)

Calcium, Vitamin D and K

Calcium is also reported to participate in melatonin secretion. (1) One study found higher calcium levels in the body provided some of the deepest sleep levels, such as the rapid eye movement phase (REM). (2)

However, without vitamin K, vitamin D and calcium can be disastrous. While vitamin D helps to absorb calcium from the intestine and circulates in the bloodstream, vitamin K helps prevent calcium from depositing in blood vessels and places it at the right place, such as bones, teeth, and other required places. Read more about this here.https://www.holistichealthnlife.com/vitamin-k2-for-heart-bone-health-benefits/

Moreover, vitamin D deficiency is associated with a higher risk of sleep disorders. (3,4)

Both vitamin K and D is needed for many vital functions.

Vitamin D food sources: (5)

Food	IUs per serving	Percent Daily value
Cod liver oil, 1 tablespoon	1,360	340
Swordfish, cooked, 3 ounces	566	142
Salmon (sockeye), cooked, 3 ounces	447	112
Tuna fish, canned in water, drained, 3 ounces	154	39
Orange juice fortified with vitamin D, 1 cup (check product labels, as the amount	137	34

Food	IUs per serving	Percent Daily value
of added vitamin D, varies)		
Milk, nonfat, reduced fat, and whole, vitamin D-fortified, 1 cup	115-124	29-31
Yogurt, fortified with 20% of the DV for vitamin D, 6 ounces (more heavily fortified yogurts provide more of the DV)	80	20
Margarine, fortified, 1 tablespoon	60	15
Sardines, canned in oil, drained, 2 sardines	46	12
Liver, beef, cooked, 3 ounces	42	11
Egg, 1 large (vitamin D is found in yolk)	41	10
Ready-to-eat cereal, fortified with 10% of the DV for vitamin D, 0.75-1 cup (more heavily fortified cereals might provide more of the DV)	40	10
Cheese, Swiss, 1 ounce	6	2

* IUs = International Units.

The upper limit for vitamin D is 1,000 to 1,500 IU/day for infants, 2,500 to 3,000 IU/day for children 1-8 years, and 4,000 IU/day for children 9 years and older, adults, and pregnant and lactating teens and women. Vitamin D toxicity almost always occurs from the overuse of supplements. Excessive sun exposure doesn't cause vitamin D poisoning because the body limits the amount of this vitamin it produces.-Source: National Institute of Health, updated as on 24 March 2020 (6)

Vitamin K food sources

Natto, egg yolk, Australian emu oil, fish, organ meat, dairy products like gouda cheese, cheese, butter, ghee, olive oil, leafy greens, and some others.

Chamomile tea

Chamomile has been used traditionally for thousands of years to calm anxiety and digestive health. Chamomile tea has shown sleep improvement in many clinical studies. Researchers believe that the antioxidant apigenin in chamomile tea binds to certain receptors in your brain that might promote sleepiness. (1)

In a study, people who consumed 270 mg of chamomile extract twice daily for 28 days had less night time awakening and fell asleep faster than those who did not take the extract. (2) In another research published in The Journal of Clinical Pharmacology, 10 out of 12 people with cardiac disease fell into a deep sleep shortly after drinking the Chamomile tea beverage. (3)

In other studies in individuals with the cardiovascular disorder and postpartum women, researchers found that drinking chamomile tea helped to fall into a deep sleep within a short period, as well as lower the symptoms of depression. (4, 5)

Other scientists also found similar results for improving sleep quality in a meta-analysis of fourteen clinical studies, as well as other clinical studies. (6, 7)

To sum up, chamomile tea before bed shows improvement in sleep in most people.

Safety of Chamomile tea

Chamomile appears safe for most people. However, some people may experience allergic reactions. Usually, these are people who have an allergy to the same plant family as ragweed, marigolds, daisies, and other related herbs. The safety of drinking chamomile tea has not been established in young children, pregnant or lactating women, and people with liver or kidney disease. Also, it is safer to check if the tea is contaminated with other harmful materials. It may have a mild blood-thinning effect, so you need to stop it in the case of any surgery ahead. (8)

Also, it is better to consume within control. And it would be better if you did not let your sleep become dependent on any single factor by making habits, including chamomile tea.

Fatty fish

Fatty fish containing vitamin D and omega 3 fatty acids may improve sleep quality by participating in serotonin synthesis. (1, 2, 3)

Although we don't have that much evidence on sleep till now, we need those nutrients. Omega 3 is an essential fatty acid that the human body can't make on its own. And vitamin D has many vital roles. In one study, men who ate 300 grams of Atlantic salmon that was a source of both vitamin D and omega 3 fatty acids three times a week for six months fell asleep about 10 minutes faster than men who ate chicken, beef, or pork. (4)

Another study suggests that the consumption of Atlantic salmon may impact mental health by regulating emotion control and reducing anxiety. Participants consumed Atlantic salmon three times per week for 23 weeks with a portion size of 150–300 g. (5)

Omega 3 fatty acids contribute to brain health and mental wellbeing, which may help with sleep. As a source of omega 3 fatty acids and vitamin D, fatty fish may improve sleep quality.

Food sources

A common source of omega3 fish oil includes herring, salmon, Pacific chub mackerel, Atlantic mackerel, Spanish mackerel, sardine, krill, crab, shrimp, etc. Due to water pollution, some fish can absorb mercury from industrial discharge. Although most fish is likely to have a small amount of mercury, some fish tend to have a higher amount. Larger predatory fish like shark, swordfish, and similar consume smaller fish and tend to have a higher level of mercury. Mercury is toxic to health, and an elevated level of mercury in the body can create serious health problems. King mackerel, bigeye tuna, and some others are identified as high-level mercury-contaminated fish. So, it is safer to search for heavy metal contaminated fish in your environment. In general, large predatory fish and fish with longer life tend to have higher mercury content. While cooking fish with omega 3, you need to be careful as eating degrades omega-3 fatty acids. Steaming and low-temperature baking are some better options for cooking such fish than frying. You should avoid high heat while cooking. Or, if you go for supplementation, be sure that the supplement is free from heavy metal contamination or molecularly distilled.

Barley grass powder

Barley grass is rich in sleep-promoting functional ingredients, such as (GABA), potassium, calcium, tryptophan, magnesium, zinc, and more. Moreover, it is also a source of health-protecting ingredients like flavonoids, primary antioxidant SOD, chlorophyll, and vitamins (A, B1, C, and E), K, dietary fiber, and some others.

According to a 2018 review, barley grass powder promotes sleep and a wide range of health-promoting effects like anti-diabetic, blood pressure regulation, enhanced immunity, liver-protecting, and anti-inflammatory antioxidant, cancer prevention, and more. (1)

Safety

Typically, people with celiac disease or other sensitivities are sensitive to barley, especially to the seed due to its gluten content. Although such sensitivity is not associated with the green leaves, you should check your health status if you are susceptible to such sensitivity.

According to drugs.com, there is no toxicology data about barley grass powder. (2) Organic and contamination-free are preferred choice as it is usually eaten in the raw state.

Lettuce

In animal studies, the seed and leaf extracts of lettuce have been shown to promote sleep. (1, 2)

In two human studies, lettuce seeds were shown to improve sleep. (3,4)

Major data about lettuce is not available.

CHAPTER 5

Macronutrients on sleep: Carbohydrates, Protein, and Fats

Fat

The role of dietary fats in sleep quality is somewhat controversial, as many studies take fats as one category, while all fats are not the same. While some studies reported improvement in sleep quality with a high-fat diet, another study indicated no relationship. (1)

A population-based study found an association between decreased sleep duration and increased fat intake. (2) Another study published in the Journal of Clinical Sleep Medicine found the intake of low fiber and high saturated fat and sugar-laden food is associated with lighter, less restorative, and more disrupted sleep. While participants who took protein and low saturated fat meal before bed fell asleep faster. (3)

On the other hand, high fat Ketogenic diets have been associated with improved sleep quality and increased REM sleep, increased slow-wave sleep, as well as less insomnia, and improved emotional functioning. (4,5,6)

Another study reported that sleep quality was significantly higher after consuming saturated and polyunsaturated fat intakes compared to sleep quality scores after consuming low-fat intakes. (7)

The problem is that there are many types of fats. Even all saturated fats are not the same. Saturated fat is a group of different types of fatty acids rather than a single type. For example, the composition of saturated fats from dairy and saturated fats from meat are not the same. There are also plant-derived saturated fats. Saturated fats are also found in many packaged foods, such as snacks, processed meats, and more. (8, 9)

What we can do is to avoid industrial trans fats, plastic or synthetic fats, rancid fats, highly processed industrial fats, high-fat snacks, fats from processed meats, or packaged foods completely. We can add saturated fats from dairy, like butter, Ghee, less processed cheese in a controlled manner, (8,9) add fats from nuts and seeds directly and from extra virgin olive oil, avocado oil, high oleic sunflower oil, and similar. Small amount of ruminant trans fat from bacterial fermentation in dairy products has no significant health concern.

Protein

You need protein for many functions. In a study, people who consumed high protein showed an increase of tryptophan in their blood circulations, an amino acid responsible for better sleep. (10)

Another study reported participants who ate protein had better sleep. (11)

Researchers also reported low protein intake (<16% of energy from protein) was associated with poor sleep quality and marginally associated with difficulty initiating sleep. In contrast, high protein intake (>19% of energy from protein) was associated with difficulty in maintaining sleep. (12)

Two clinical studies on overweight adults found that those on a 20% and 30% protein diet had a better sleep than a 10% protein diet. (13)

For adults, the present RDA for protein is 0.8 g/kg, representing the minimum intake needed to prevent malnutrition.

On the other hand, Layman et al. estimate that protein requirements at ~1.2 g per kg per day are beneficial for various metabolic functions. (14)

Nancy Rodriguez, a registered dietitian and professor of nutritional science at the University of Connecticut in Storrs estimates roughly 15% to 25% of protein of total daily calories, although it could be above or below this range, depending on your age, sex, and activity level. Rodriguez was among more than 40 nutrition scientists who gathered in Washington, D.C., for a "Protein Summit" to discuss research on protein and human health. This was published in Harvard Health Publishing at the Harvard Medical School. (15)

A statistical analysis of the data used to establish the RDA suggests this number should be higher: 1.0 g/kg. (16)

Research on the optimal amount of protein for good health is ongoing and appears far from settled. The intake of protein also depends on physical activity level, age, and sex. What can we do? We can consider RDA protein as 0.8 g/kg as minimum intake to prevent malnutrition and can increase this to an extent, depending on physical activities. However, before having a considerably higher amount, you should consult your healthcare professional.

Protein should be from healthier choices, whether it's a well-balanced toxin-free plant protein or hormone, antibiotic, or other toxin-free meat sources.

Carbohydrates

Researchers found a high glycemic diet of carbohydrates with less fiber; processed foods can lead to sleep disturbance. (17)

The quality of carbohydrates is more important than the quantity. In a modern lifestyle with less physical activities, simple carbohydrates with a high glycemic load can create metabolic problems. Usually, carbohydrates that go several stages before coming to your plate are high glycemic, simple carbohydrates. In opposite foods in their natural state are mostly complex carbohydrates and low glycemic scores except for some foods. Carbohydrates with low glycemic load release sugar into the bloodstream in a controlled manner.

On the other hand, high glycemic diet carbohydrates suddenly increase blood sugar. Whole foods and minimally processed foods are better choices than highly processed foods, snacks, sugar-sweetened foods, and beverages. While whole foods and minimally processed foods retain most of their natural nutrients package, highly processed foods don't.

To sum up

To sum up, pairing a limited amount of protein, more specifically protein-containing tryptophan, with complex carbohydrates containing fiber or good fats(in low amount) at night can help for better sleep. Dietary fiber is good for many reasons. You can have a considerable amount of dietary fiber from vegetables, whole grain, and fruits. However, if you have conditions like SIBO, bacterial overgrowth, or IBD or IBS, then too much fiber intake may worsen the situation.

Therefore, consult your healthcare provider before taking high fiber foods that may increase your intake.

Consuming tryptophan and a carbohydrate-rich, protein-poor meal increases brain levels of tryptophan and serotonin. Although a carbohydrate meal itself lacks tryptophan, the meal causes insulin to be secreted. Insulin, in turn, decreases plasma levels of large neutral amino acids that would ordinarily compete with tryptophan for transport across the blood-brain barrier. (18, 19)

In short, carbohydrates make tryptophan more available in the brain that helps you sleep better, while eating large protein meals may compete with tryptophan. As we have discussed earlier, a set of complex carbohydrates with moderate protein and foods with tryptophan makes it easy.

Similarly, studies also indicated good quality fats could improve sleep. (20) Making a balance, rather than depending on a single nutrient is more important.

CHAPTER 6

Nighttime foods that can steal your sleep

Stop having coffee or tea or caffeine foods in the evening, and instead of Coffee and tea....

We know that our body breaks down glucose into Adenosine Tri-Phosphate (ATP) to use as energy. When your body uses ATP for energy, adenosine is produced, which diffuses from cells to interact with adenosine receptors. (1, 2)

Apart from other biochemical functions, adenosine also acts as a central nervous system neuromodulator. It has specific roles in sleep regulation. When adenosine binds to its receptors, it slows down neural activity, and you feel and tired sleepy. (3, 4, 5, 6)

That means after a period of energy expenditure, adenosine level increases, binds with its receptors, and signals you to sleep. Remember, your body uses energy even you are sitting on a chair.

Stimulants like Coffee, tea contain caffeine in varying amounts. Even green tea also contains some amount of caffeine. Caffeine causes most of its biological effects via antagonizing all types of adenosine receptors. (7) That's why Coffee and tea or similar that contain caffeine can help you to perform some cognitive task even if you have less sleep the last night. They help in low levels of wakefulness and thus help you to complete some cognitive tasks. However, it may produce detrimental effects on subsequent sleep. (8)

Therefore, if you have a drink with caffeine in the evening, it will negatively impact your sleep at night. The disruptive sleep effects of caffeine intake at bedtime are well-documented. In a study on healthy day workers, researchers found that people who took caffeine 0, 3, or even 6 hours before bedtime had sleep disruption and reduced total sleep time. (9, 10)

Avoid stimulants like Coffee, tea that contains caffeine in the evening, as they will impact your sleep.

What can we take instead of tea or Coffee in the evening?

I prefer a cup of caffeine-free infusions like basil, ginger, or peppermint in the evening if necessary. (11)

Basil and ginger also possess stress-relieving properties. (12, 13, 14, 15)

A study suggested that peppermint oil also helps to relieve stress. (16)

According to a review published in the Journal of Pharmaceutical Sciences & Research, peppermint is good for stress relief. (17)

The National Sleep Foundation also recommended ginger and peppermint tea as calming choices for bedtime. (18)

 So, these stress relievers help to drain some amount of your daily stress in the evening. It is better to choose good quality and have in a controlled manner. I prefer to keep different infusions in my cupboard and take what I like most at that moment.

Besides Coffee, some other foods also contain a higher amount of caffeine

Apart from Coffee and tea, some common foods or drinks, such as dark chocolate, diet soda, chocolate cake with frosting, also may contain caffeine in varying amounts. Besides these energy drinks, breakfast cereals, or similar, with an attempt to energy boost may also have caffeine. Other such as ice cream, frozen yogurt, pudding, or similar may also have caffeine or chocolate punch. (19, 20)

Foods that contain high tyramine

Amino acid Tyramine is thought to promote blood pressure elevation. Moreover, it may constrict blood vessels in the brain, resulting in migraine attacks in susceptible persons. (21,22)

According to WebMD, tyramine is a well-accepted migraine trigger. (23)

Although there is not much study, a double-blind clinical trial found that people with migraine required significantly less tyramine to increase their systolic blood pressure by 30 mm Hg when compared with matched controls. (24) That means even a lesser amount of tyramine can increase blood pressure in migraines than healthy.

Enzyme monoamine oxidase (MAO) breaks down excess tyramine in the body and helps to excrete it. According to the Mayo Clinic, a high intake of tyramine with medications called monoamine oxidase inhibitors (MAOIs) can cause a serious elevation in blood pressure and require emergency action. (25)

Foods, especially aged and fermented foods, contain higher tyramine percentages.

Some common food that may contain high tyramine(26)

Cheese and dairy foods

While aged cheese contains a higher amount of tyramine, fresh dairy and some dairy products contain lower amounts.

Higher in tyramine: Aged cheeses like cheddar, Stilton or blue, Camembert, Swiss, feta, Muenster, Parmesan

Lower in tyramine: American cheese, cottage cheese, yogurt, fresh milk, farmer's cheese, cream cheese, sour cream.

The National Sleep Foundation recommended cottage cheese, which contains amino acid tryptophan, which helps to sleep better. To make it more attractive, you can also add some raspberries, which are a rich source of the sleep hormone melatonin. (27)

Meat, poultry, and fish

Foods high in protein may contain more tyramine if they have been stored for a long time and/or not been kept cold enough. Smoked fish, cured meat, etc. can typically have a higher amount of tyramine. Fresh meat like poultry, fish, eggs contains a comparatively lower amount of tyramine.

Fruits, veggies, and beans

Some plant-based foods also contain a higher percentage of tyramine.

Higher in tyramine: oranges, grapefruit, lemons, limes, tangerines, pineapple, fava beans, broad beans, raw onions, etc. Fermented foods like sauerkraut, fermented soy foods, miso, tofu, kimchee, Low in tyramine: Most fresh, frozen veggies

Drinks or beverages

Alcoholic beverages like Vermouth, some types of beers, red wine contain a higher amount of tyramine.

Condiments

Concentrated yeast extract, sauces like soy sauce, fish sauce, teriyaki sauce, etc. may contain a higher amount of tyramine.

Smoked, aged, pickled, or fermented foods generally may contain a higher amount of tyramine. Such foods need to be refrigerated and should be consumed within a shorter period. If you feel such foods impair your sleep, it is better to say no to such foods at night.

Foods with a diuretic effect

Some foods are naturally diuretic. Diuretics increase the amount of urine you produce and help to excrete excess water. Thus, diuretics help to reduce extra water content in the body. However, taking food with a high diuretic effect before bed may increase urination and wake you up in the night. Some such foods with higher diuretic effects are Coffee, green tea, black tea, watermelon, grapes, berries, celery, onion, asparagus, bell pepper, cucumber, beetroots, citrus food like lemon, and some more. (28, 29, 30)

A small amount may not have much effect; however, having a large amount may interrupt your sleep.

Avoid a large meal before bed

If you eat a large meal before bed, your digestion will slow, which may lead to indigestion and impaired metabolism. That can make you uncomfortable and may also interrupt your sleep. Moreover, you will store excess energy as fat, as during sleep, you are not using that much energy. A night of good sleep is restorative to your health. Therefore if your body is busy with digestion, the restorative process can be impaired. (31, 32)

Similarly, taking too much fluid before bed can cause excessive urination and sleep interruption. (33)

A study published in the Journal of Clinical Sleep Medicine found that low fiber and high-fat and sugar-filled snacks and meals before bed are associated with lighter, less restorative, and more disrupted sleep. While participants who took protein and low-fat meal before bed reportedly fell asleep faster. (34)

A high-fat diet in the night may impair sleep at night. And sugar-laden foods are definitely a no.

Deep-fried foods

Deep-frying with low grade cooking oil and reheated oils often releases higher level toxic aldehydes. Although some are volatile, others remain after frying and can be found in cooked food. Aldehydes are believed to be related to some neurodegenerative diseases and some types of cancer. (35)

Moreover, such food can cause inflammation inside your body and can also cause heartburn. Any other food that can upset your stomach can also interrupt your sleep.

Does alcohol help you to sleep better?

Does alcohol before bed help to have a better sleep? Some may tell you –I have a drink and sleep better. If alcohol helps you sleep better, then why do you have a hangover the next day? Alcohol interferes with brain signals and inhibits the release of the signaling molecule (i.e., neurotransmitter). Researchers also reported acute alcohol consumption activates brain reward by releasing the feel-good hormone dopamine. (36)

Probably due to that reason, some people feel less stressed with alcohol consumption. However, the problem is that if a factor continuously stimulates dopamine, it becomes less responsive to that factor. (37)

That means you will need more alcohol intake to have the same pleasing effect if you consume it day by day. Moreover, damage to brain cells is associated with alcohol use disorder. (38)

 Alcohol may help induce sleep, and you sleep deeply for a while, but overall, it can cause disruptive sleep. It reduces rapid eye movement (REM) sleep. REM sleep occurs about 90 minutes after we fall asleep. In this stage of sleep, people dream, and it's thought to be restorative. Disruptions in REM sleep may cause daytime drowsiness and poor concentration. (39) Moreover, alcohol has been shown to reduce the production of the sleep hormone melatonin. (40)

To sum up, we found that although alcohol may induce sleep in the initial stage, it causes disruptive sleep in the later stage. (40)Due to such disruption in sleep, you feel hungover the next day. Drinking more closure to bedtime more negatively affects sleep.

Update: A recent cross-sectional study among 4050 individuals published in the Journal of American Medical Association in July 2020 concluded decreased percentage REM sleep was associated with greater risk of all-cause, cardiovascular, and other non-cancer-related mortality. (41)

CHAPTER 7

Gut health

Gut health affects nearly every aspect of human health, including mental health. That's why gut health is vital. The human body is a resident of a dynamic population of microorganisms, such as bacteria, fungi, and viruses that live together in a harmonic and dynamic equilibrium. Some microorganisms are friendly, some are harmful, and some may be neutral. There are so many varieties that researchers are yet to understand them all. When pathogenic microorganisms overpower the friendly or there is an imbalance of microorganisms, many health problems begin. Those microorganisms are major bacteria and mostly reside in the gut. The number of microorganisms inhabiting the Gastro-intestinal tract has been estimated to exceed 100 trillion, which encompasses ~10 times more bacterial cells than the number of human cells. (1)

A 2017 systematic review of 10 clinical studies assessed the effects of probiotics intake on mood, anxiety, and cognition. Scientists found that most of the studies had positive results in alleviating symptoms and improving mental health. (2)

Friendly bacterial culture or probiotics promote health in wide ways, along with restoring gut health. Probiotic foods, such as kefir, yogurt or curd, kimchi, etc. with friendly bacterial culture promote gut health, reduce gut inflammation and diseases. (3, 4, 5,6, 7)

Some fermented foods like kefir, yogurt, kimchi, curd, etc. can be made at home by learning how to make them. Kefir and yogurt cultures are available in the market and easy to prepare at home by buying good cultures from stores. These cultures are also available at large online stores. Similarly, kimchi is also not difficult to make if you know how to make it. Purchasing live cultured such probiotic foods is not always available in the store. Many times, cultures die during processing, transportation, and harsh storage environment. Some manufacturers may use technology to keep their culture alive. For that reason, unsweetened live-cultured yogurt, kefir, or kimchi is preferable.

There are also other fermented foods with a bacterial culture like unsweetened curd, kombucha tea, tempeh, sauerkraut, pickled fruits and vegetables, cultured condiments, etc. (8, 9)

Otherwise, an excellent probiotic supplement helps to restore and maintain the gut bacterial ecosystem. However, if you are critically ill, don't use probiotics and also consult with your healthcare provider with knowledge on the subject before supplementation.

On the other hand, foods with prebiotics or dietary fiber pass through the small intestine mostly undigested. These are fermented in the large intestine by gut microflora. This process generally promotes the growth of the friendly bacteria in your gut and helps them to produce essential nutrients in return. (10, 11, 12)

Mostly plant-based foods contain varying amounts of fiber with a higher amount in foods like beans or legumes, whole grains, and other vegetables and fruits. Apart from those, some foods that contain a considerable amount of prebiotics include artichoke, asparagus, edible mushrooms, leeks, garlic, onion, cabbage, banana, apple, grapefruits, watermelon, nuts & seeds, marine foods like seaweed, and more.

More is always not better. As we talked earlier, too much fiber in the diet may increase gastrointestinal symptoms, especially in conditions like SIBO, IBS, and IBD. (13) We have talked about this earlier. Foods belonging to FODMAPs like beans and legumes are commonly intolerable in such cases.

Apart from these, regular forest walking or spending some time with the natural environment also helps to shape the bacterial ecosystem. (14, 15)

The gut restoration process takes several processes, like following an autoimmune paleo diet and restricting hard digestible foods, allergic foods, sugar-laden foods, and similar for a period. Supplements with probiotics, glutamine, foods with zinc, restoring stomach acid should be followed. Then slowly re-introduce foods in a controlled manner and identify foods that cause an allergic reaction and eliminate those permanently.

However, this book is not aimed to heal the gut. If you want to know more about gut healing strategies, read Dr. Michael Ruscio "Healthy Gut, Healthy You: The Personalized Plan to Transform Your Health from the Inside Out." This book has wonderful information, and Dr.Ruscio provides strategies about different stages of gut health. I am not affiliated or endorsed with this book. I have just mentioned as I found it is a good book.

CHAPTER 8

Effect of light, color, temperature, and noise in Bedroom

Color-light

The color of light significantly affects sleep. Research has shown that blue light suppresses melatonin, impacts the circadian clock, and increases alertness. Also, Light-Emitting eReaders before bedtime can adversely affect sleep. Many light-emitting eReaders, tablets, laptops, cell phones, LED monitors, and other electronic devices, emit blue light. Overall, reducing exposure to blue light before sleep or avoiding blue light in the Bedroom can help for better sleep.

According to Harvard Health Publishing, even dim light can interfere with a person's circadian rhythm and melatonin secretion. While the light of any kind can suppress melatonin's secretion, blue light at night does this so more powerfully. LED lights also produce a fair amount of light in the blue spectrum. They suggest avoiding looking at bright screens beginning two to three hours before bed. Night workers can wear blue-blocking glasses or install an app that filters the blue/green wavelength at night. (1, 2)

Exposure to such a light-emitting screen can delay your sleep. Some people argue that they eat lots of rice, take the cell-phone and fall asleep after some time. This might be due to the rice, as rice consumers were reported to have a good sleep. Researchers found an association of good sleep with rice consumption in a study on 1,848 Japanese men and women between 20 and 60 years of age. (3)

On the negative side, white rice has a high glycemic load that increases your blood sugar and calls insulin for action. In modern sedentary life, excessive stimulation of insulin can lead to numerous health disorders like obesity, diabetes, heart disease, and many more. If you are not involved in physical activities, consuming too much rice can create problems for you.

To sum up, blue light and other bright light delays sleep. Avoid such light two hours before sleep. In the case of a computer, tablet, and mobile phone, or similar, you can use a light-blocking screen. Make your Bedroom dark enough. If you are not comfortable with complete darkness, you may use low-intensity dim light only. You can also consider sleep musk for eyes.

Noise

Noise can drastically interrupt your sleep and also increase the time taken to fall asleep. If external noise enters your Bedroom, make it soundproof. Also, you may try a comfortable earplug if your Bedroom is exposed to noise.

Alternatively, you can try a good white noise machine that can help to mask external noise that can potentially disturb your sleep.

The TV volume also raises the noise level. Some people like soothing music, but the volume needs to be kept low.

Use of smart gadgets

Amazon's new generation Echo dot has voice recognition ability. Alexa adapts to your speech patterns and vocabulary. You can use the Echo dot to play music, call Alexa to switch off your bedroom light if you feel sleepy and don't want to get out of your bed. I am not affiliated with the Echo dot with this writing.

But don't forget, too much use of gadgets may make you lazy. Always use them in a positive way.

Bedroom temperature

If the bedroom temperature is not comfortable enough, it may interrupt your sleep and wake you up.

According to *the National Sleep Foundation*, in general, the suggested bedroom temperature should be between 60 and 67 degrees Fahrenheit or 16 degrees Celsius and 19 degrees Celsius for optimal sleep. For a baby or toddler, raising the thermostat a little higher between 65 and 70 degrees will suffice. (4)

Also, the temperature at which a person feels comfortable may be different for others. However, a too cold or too hot bedroom temperature can negatively affect sleep.

Overall, your Bedroom should be quiet, cool, dark enough, and comfortable enough to make you relax and sleep well. (4)

CHAPTER 9

Activities that can hurt your sleep

Stop naps after 3 pm

A short daytime sleep helps to boost brainpower. However, you should avoid taking naps after 3 pm as this can make it harder to fall asleep at night. (1)

Bedtime use of cell phone/tablets

We are living in a world full of gadgets. Gadgets help us in many ways but also harm some ways. So, the right use of devices is very much essential. Unfortunately, many of us are not realizing that the bedtime use of cell phones and tablets can steal our sleep, a small fact but a big impact. And there is more than a single reason for how cell phone takes our sleep.

Reason one- suppress the secretion of the sleep hormone melatonin

We know that the hormone melatonin tells us to go to sleep. We talked-while lights of any kind can suppress the secretion of the sleep hormone melatonin, blue light at night does so more powerfully. The blue light emitted by screens on cell phones, computers, tablets, and televisions restrain melatonin production and disrupt circadian rhythm. With the suppression of melatonin, you need a longer time to fall asleep. (1, 2, 3, 4, 5)

Reason two-keep your mind engaged

The use of smart-phones makes our life more informative, productive, and also provides entertainment. But it is now time to sleep and keep everything aside. Checking emails or social media can keep our minds engaged many times. Message from the mail, social media (binge-watching in social media can show both good and unpleasant notes) can chew our emotions. And our idea of answering can keep our sleep at bay. (3, 6, 7)

Reason three-disrupt REM sleep and tired & less alert the next day

REM or Rapid Eye Movement phase of sleep consolidates memories and is tied to your creative and problem-solving skills. Not having REM sleep, it can leave you feeling groggy and having difficulty concentrating the next day. According to the Cleveland Clinic, emotions can trigger a response that prolongs falling sleep, which consequently delays REP sleep.

Such gadgets delay the onset of REM sleep, reduce the total amount of REM sleep, and compromise alertness the next morning. Over time, these effects can add up to a significant, chronic deficiency in sleep-The National Sleep Foundation explained. (6, 7, 8, 9)

Many sleep and health authorities warn about bedtime exposure to such gadgets.

Should you do exercise before bedtime?

Mostly, exercises in the daytime improve daytime activeness and night-time sleep. However, should you do exercise before bed?

There is some belief that vigorous bouts of late-night exercise can lead to sleep difficulty. Exercising raises your core body temperature, increases your heart rate, and prompts your system to release stimulating hormone epinephrine (adrenaline). The brain becomes more active with such exercise, adrenaline is high, and it needs time to cool down. (1)

What should be the time gap between exercise and bedtime?

To evaluate this, Sports Medicine published a systematic review of 23 studies in 2019 on the effects of Evening Exercise on Sleep in Healthy Participants. They concluded that the reviewed studies do not support the hypothesis that evening exercise negatively affects sleep; in fact, rather the opposite. However, those who did vigorous exercise less than one hour before bedtime took a longer time to fall asleep and had poorer sleep quality. (2, 3)

In fact, a 2016 published review of multiple studies found meditative movements like tai chi, qi gong, and yoga had beneficial effects on the improvement of sleep. They found improvement in sleep quality in the majority of studies, along with improvements in quality of life, physical performance, and depression. (4)

Doing exercise is always better than not doing-if you can. Vigorous exercise needs to be avoided at least one hour before bed. Instead, a meditative movement like yoga, Pilates, tai chi, meditation, or simple stretching can be tried before bed for better sleep. (5)

However, if you feel trouble with exercise, it is better to wait some hours between exercise and bedtime.

How good is watching TV before bed for sleep?

While plenty of people watch TV before bed, many health authorities recommend no exposure to your eyes on a screen before bed. While blue light or even a dim light can interfere with a person's circadian rhythm and melatonin secretion at night, watching TV also suppress melatonin secretion. Even LED lights also may produce a fair amount of light in the blue spectrum. (1, 2)

One study showed suppression in melatonin among people who used screens in the hours before bed. (3)

It creates even more stress to your eye if you are watching a screen in a dark room.

Another problem with watching bedtime TV is simply the temptation to stay up late to find out what happens next. Additionally, violence, a bloody show, or suspense may leave you feeling anxious. But in reality, most of these are not the concern. Similarly, some shows may trigger your emotions and make you panic. (4)

But other situations also exist

Watching TV before bed is not encouraged; however, in some way, watching TV can provide some relaxing aids if used in some other way. Many times, a racing brain overloaded with activities, multi-tasking is very disturbing. You try to close your eyes, and your brain is scrolling through what you have done wrong or what is going to be wrong. This may be even worse if you are living alone.

That can create pain, anxiety and steal your sleep when you try to close your eyes. And a TV show with violence, emotional triggers, a lot of noise with loudness even may bombard your unstable mind. But in some other way, watching TV can aid some remedies in such a situation. Plenty of people also tune the TV in an attempt to be relaxed.

 For example, if you are overloaded with a whole day's stress and want to re-watch some of your low noise favorites, then there is something interesting. A TV episode or movie that you've already seen several times can offer a sense of familiarity and comfort and won't pull your emotional response, which may help to minimize the negativity of the mind. And that helps to calm you down.

In a study, researchers found watching a re-run of a favorite show restored their energy levels. However, binge-watching doesn't have the same effect. (5)

Another point that makes a difference from using a smart-phone or computer with TV is, while you are using a smart-phone, tablet, or computer, your eyes are close to the screen, while typically, the TV screen stays a few feet away. A study found that computer use increases the risk of poor sleep among university students while watching TV during the same periods did not present the same risk. (6)

Watching TV before bed all depends on the person. For some, it may be preferable to watch TV to calm anxiety, then switch off the TV, and sleep. For some people, it may work.

Reading a book with cool thoughts is a better option. Many times, a good book works as a good friend and can give you positive thoughts. Alternatively, rather than taking a meal and immediately switching on the TV, have a walk or spend some time with relaxing activities with family, friends, or pets and then go and watch the TV. Keep in mind that the TV show is not triggering your sense of emotion. You can automatically set the timer down the TV after one hour or use a smart gadget like a new generation Amazon echo dot. You may also try a screen blue light & glare filter. But also make sure you don't become too dependent on TV to use as a sleep aid, and spending hours in front of the TV is not a healthier choice. According to the National Sleep Foundation, even though you might feel like you can fall asleep just fine after your show, the exposure to blue light can delay the onset of REM sleep and lead to morning drowsiness. (7)

Watching TV before bed is a topic of debate. And we don't have many scientific studies. Sometimes, I watch some low noise programs like geographic or Earth channels, History, health, and cooking. Such channels don't sue my emotion and increase anxiety. Whether I watch TV before bedtime or not depends on that particular time. However, it may not be the same may with you. I act differently after dinner to break monotonous ways. It is perhaps better to figure out what works for you more healthily. And if you do not need to watch TV to fall asleep, then don't go for it. Or even if watching TV helps you to fall asleep, don't make this a habit.

Eliminate electromagnetic fields (EMFs) from your Bedroom

There is some indication of the effect of electromagnetic waves on the brain. (1, 2)It is better to eliminate electromagnetic waves from your Bedroom. If possible, switch off your mobile phone or otherwise you can keep it in a separate room.

CHAPTER 10

Strategies for going to bed

Clam down your racing mind

With the whole day's workload, your mind still is running with your daily activities at night; it's time to calm down your mind. Prepare yourself, your body, your mind for a good sleep.

Make a note of activities for the next day.

Maintain a notebook and note down all the planning for the next day or week a few hours before bed. That will help to reduce the load on your brain, clear your mind, and you'll feel more relaxed. Organize your activities and get in the habit of making a to-do list according to priority. If you have work to do, you need to have an idea about what you are going to do the next morning. Otherwise, it will be a confused state of mind. Have a realistic goal, and find a way to perform and do them within the limit. We will talk more about this in the goal-setting strategies.

Also, don't forget to review periodically to check progress or for any change if needed. Without reviewing, some essential tasks may leave out, building in a pile and developing stress. A periodical review is essential.

Turn off your computer, email, social profile

Shut off your computer at least 90 minutes before sleep and indulge yourself in something peaceful and pleasurable. Similarly, also keep the smart-phone away from you 90 minutes before sleep. You are not using, but keeping a smart-phone within reach can still disturb you. The smart-phone can be a stressor, a media to make your life measurable many times. In the work-lives of some peoples, they are using cell-phone for late nights. However, there is no such emergency in most cases; instead, it is created as an emergency. If you want to avoid such a situation, you may simply don't respond well to such calls or tell to talk the next day. After a few days, your night-time calls from work-life may go down. Alternatively, you can have your own personal number for the absolute use of phone calls.

Checking mail or social media on a smart-phone can hijack your thoughts, and your mind may indulge in those thinking. Often, messages in mail or social media messages are not very pleasurable and have enough power to fix your thoughts. Mostly, the Artificial Intelligence of social media is designed to fix your thoughts and make you alert using notifications. Many people (not all) built a habit of checking their smart-phones every few minutes. Take control over gadgets; don't let gadgets to control you.

A study among 1788 young adults published in the journal Preventive Medicine found that the more people used social media (in general, not just before/in bed) had significantly greater odds of having sleep disturbance. (1)

Another study among 1763 adults found social media use for just 30 minutes before bed is independently associated with disturbed sleep. (2)

It is true that social media is now our part of life. So, if you watch social media, keep a separate time to manage social media and emails rather than checking short intervals.

Your Bedroom should be a place for relaxation, rest, love, and sex.

The start and end of a day

While organizing activities for the next day or the week with a realistic goal helps to relieve the load from your mind before sleep, healthily starting the day is equally important.

Similarly, never start the day by checking your email or social media. What will happen if you start the day by checking mail or social media? For example, you check your social media account, and you will see some likes-comments that give you some pleasure, but you will also see some posts or comments that you dislike and are pulling all your thoughts and emotions. You check the mail and found some emails you don't expect, and it starts pulling your thoughts. You planned to do something last night, but now your mind is running with some new thoughts, and you haven't enough idea right now on what to do. What you had organized to do is now in the back seat. And your unfinished works are now beginning to pile up. Those things have enough power to divert you from your focus so that you don't get your job done and put you in a stressful situation. It's is very important to start the day positively. Wake up in the morning, open the window, make the bed, be fresh, and let the fresh air come in. Start with one action; don't try multiple activities at a time. You can try it for a few days and feel the differences.

Get up in the morning; let the sunlight to fall on your face. That will stop your melatonin secretion and prepare you for the day. Starting the day with 20-30 minutes of exercise, yoga, or meditation gives a positive kick start for the day and makes you feel better for the day, and helps you sleep better at night. We will know more why this is so important in the exercise part.

These small things have a significant impact on health as well as in life. Unfortunately, many (not all) of us don't realize this and become addicted to gadgets.

Candlelight dinner

Many people find that a candlelight dinner is more calming than dinner in bright light. Imagine how you will feel when you have a candlelight dinner with your family or friends with a free mind.

Don't go to bed if you don't feel tired and need sleep

Staying in bed but not falling asleep for a long time is not a good idea. Instead, do something that gives you pleasure and calms down your racing mind.

Pssseggiata-Leisure walking

In Italy, people used to walk or stroll mostly in the evening. It is mainly for socializing for pleasure. But that gives dual benefits, stress-relieving fun and some physical activities. Try it for 20 minutes after dinner with your friend, neighbors, or pet. Enjoy the moment, forget your fitness band or other activity trackers, don't put in mechanical activity, have pleasure, and let it flow naturally. It can help you to digest your food, relax your mind. Do whatever best suits you.

A warm bath before sleep

A warm bath before bed can help to relax you. Moreover, after a bath, your body temperature starts dropping, which allows you to sleep better. But what time before bed should you take a bath?

To find out, researchers conducted a Meta-analysis of studies and published them in the journal of Sleep Medicine Reviews in 2019. In collaboration with the UT Health Science Center at Houston and the University of Southern California, the UT researchers analyzed and searched through a total of 5,322 studies from databases, such as PubMed, CINAHL, Cochran, Medline, PsycInfo, and Web of Science.

They analyzed the effects of water-based passive body heating on several sleep-related factors: how long it takes to fall asleep from wakefulness, total sleep time; the amount of time spent asleep relative to the total amount of time spent in bed in an attempt to sleep; subjective sleep quality, etc. And finally, as a result of the analysis, researchers found that the best time for taking a shower or a bath is 1–2 hours before going to bed. They also indicated that a bath or shower duration need not be more than 10 minutes to reduce the time to fall asleep. Warm baths and showers stimulate the body's thermoregulatory system. That causes an increase in blood circulation from the internal core of the body to other sites, such as the hands and feet, resulting in efficient removal of body heat, and, as a result, body temperature drops. (3,4,5)

Reading a book

Reading can be a wonderful way to escape from everyday stress at the end of the day. Those who have a habit of reading can understand this.

A 2009 study found that just a few minutes of reading reduced stress by 68%. It works better and faster than other relaxing methods like listening to music or a cup of tea. That helps to clear the mind and free from the stressors that plague your daily life. If you are struggling with sleep, reading a good book before sleep can help you beyond relaxation. The habit of good reading helps to improve cognitive benefits, protect against dementia, and promote wellbeing. (6,7,8,9)

The National Sleep Foundation suggests reading an old-fashioned, printed book under lamplight. However, a phone, tablet, or laptop that emits specific light can suppress melatonin release and induce difficulty in fall asleep. However, eBooks like Kindle Paper-white, with specialized technology designed to mimic the appearance of ink on paper and traditional print books, are better options than a phone or tablet that emits light. Also, keep in mind that the book's plot is not so exciting that it ignites your mind. (10)

Meditation

Meditation helps to calm down the racing mind. We will discuss why it is so important and talk about a meditation technique in our wellbeing chapter.

Soothing sound

Listening music, soothing sound are some relaxing therapy that helps to calm you down. Choose what helps you to calm down and relax. You can also listen to your favorite podcast recording.

Wearing socks during bedtime

If you live in a cold region or in winter, wearing socks helps you sleep better. According to the National Sleep Foundation, when you warm your cold feet before sleep causes dilation of the blood vessels—which may tell the brain that it is bedtime. Wearing a suitable pair of socks to warm cold feet may be a smart way to speed up your trip to dreamland. (11)

Avoid compression socks unless and until your doctor prescribes them.

Alternatively, you could have a warm bath.

Probably most of us know that uncontrollable stress can change our behavior, cause pain in our lives. Most of us are living a busy, stressful life. That has an impact on our overall experience, including sleep, eating behaviour or the choice of foods. We will discuss strategies that we can apply to cope with stress next and later for wellbeing. We will also talk about the importance of exercise in balancing hormones that controls our mood and feeling good. And we will have some simple strategies to do exercise in our busy lives.

CHAPTER 11

Stress handling

Findings from a review paper published in the journal of Experimental Neurobiology evidenced stress-related sleep disorders lead to a vicious circle in both physiological and behavioral responses. (1) Cardiovascular disease, obesity, diabetes, depression, anxiety, impaired immune function, headaches, pain, and sleep problems are some of the documented health problems associated with stress. (2)

Stress is an inevitable part of everyone's life. We can't escape from stress. We also need some amount of stress in life. Otherwise, life will be boring. It goes wrong when stress becomes uncontrollable and chronic. Chronic uncontrollable stress impairs our cognitive decision, our emotional behavior, harm our health, including change of food selection. In modern days, too much workload, excessive busyness can create havoc in the lives of many. Sometimes you may feel that life is totally dark and gone away from you; then, you are not alone in this world. Don't let you down, don't beat yourself. It is time to rethink, think from outside the box.

The fact is that it matters more how we respond to our stressors rather than what the stress is. Remember, everyone responds to the same stressor differently. Some go down to a stressful situation, while some others take that as a positive challenge. You will see examples of many people who rise from zero from an extremely stressful situation. And it is you who will decide which path you need to choose in response to a stressful situation. It is time to rethink outside the box from a broader perspective. Horrible conditions are not permanent. There is pain behind every success. Often, a stressful situation kicks us from a dull life to a better direction; we realize that later in our lives.

The wise use of our emotions matters a lot. It is important to pay more attention to what matters most and pay less to those that matter less.

Some small adjustments in our work-life can give a direction that many times we forget to understand. So, we will talk about some strategies here. I am not going to talk too much, just going to have some brief discussion. Many times combined effects of different stressors can make us feel bad. If we can reduce some of them, the net result will be a much lower stress level.

In this part, we will discuss some stress handling strategies, and shortly we will talk about wellbeing strategy. I am going to brief.

Some strategies I had learned from an article in helpguide.org written by Lawrence Robinson, Melinda Smith, M.A., and Robert Segal, M.A. (3)

Avoiding non-essential stress

Although it is not always a good idea to avoid stress, it is better to avoid some if there is too much unnecessary stressor. If there are lots of stresses pinning you, it may make your stress level uncontrollable. You need to understand what is important for you what is not. When you understand that, it is better to avoid some of the unnecessary stress. How can you prevent the un-necessary stressor?

Make a choice-Learn to say No

Taking responsibility for everything can make you stressed. Moreover, participating in a too-much activity doesn't give better results. Accepting what you can do and what you can't do can relieve lots of stress. Earlier, I was also a victim of such behavior.

And acknowledge what you have chosen and accept the responsibility.

Avoid some kind of talking/peoples

Avoid peoples or talking that negatively affects you. If someone is frequently causing stress to you negatively, avoid such person or at least limit your time spending with such person.

Taking control over the negative environment

Negative environments exist in all of our lives. It depends on how we can handle such situations. For example-if TV news makes you anxious, don't start the day with news and similarly don't watch before bed. Choose a convenient time to watch the news. If external noise is disturbing, you use an earplug or headphone to enjoy your favorite music; if road traffic irritates you, use a different route. Many times messages in social media interrupt your thoughts and work. You need to figure out what will work for you.

Altering stressful situation

Another way to manage stressful situations is altering the stressful situation.

Express your feelings to a stressful situation

If you are not agreed with something, don't be shy and keep the load. Express your feeling gently. For example, If you are doing some serious task and someone is bothering you, say that you can only a few minutes talk or talk later. If you don't express your voice, that can continue, and the stress will increase.

Compromising with a situation

Many times a situation is ended up with a compromised decision. That also can be positive. You also are willing to change something of yours if you ask someone to change their behavior.

Adapting stress

Reframe problems in the right perspective

With every problem, there is a positive side also. When a situation is tempted by a cognitive distortion— such as thinking one mistake could ruin the whole career — positive-minded people respond by reframing the message they give themselves. Opportunity comes with a problem. Many times we don't see. It would help if you calmed yourself down with some activities that you can enjoy and come out of the situation. Review later the situation from a bigger picture, what you can lose, what you can gain.

Again I like to tell you it is much worthy of spending a few minutes calmly, uninterrupted for your own to rethink outside the box from a broader perspective to figure it out. Close your eyes, take a deep breath, aware of your body, aware of your soul, and rethink. Note down at least the common stressors in your life, like

- What is the root cause of stress
- How it affects you emotionally, physically along with eating behavior
- How you are responding to them
- Identify your resources, strength, weakness, negative emotions and the surroundings
- Make an action plan, how you can do to overcome it or feel yourself better, and move forward
- How you are feeling after an alteration of a thing or building a good habit

Sometimes a solution may not come in a single day. This is the truth for most of us. Look at the big picture, like what will happen after a few months. Apart from the gain or loss, such situations allow personal growth. Positive-minded people use healthy activities, like going for a walk or participating in a hobby, or attending a healthy social event to cope with emotional pain. But they also reserve time to be alone with their thoughts. They choose to use stressful circumstances as an opportunity to become stronger and better.

Adjust your standards

Perfectionism is another common source of stress that you can manage. Many times a task can't be completed in an attempt to be perfect, and anxiety starts to develop. But the truth is that in many times we can come forward without being wrong and perfection. And perfection is nearly impossible most of the time for the hard things.

Accept that stress as part of life.

If changing the stressor is not your hand, then you can adapt to the situation by adjusting yourself. You may need to change your attitude, your expectation to cope up with the situation. It just depends on how you respond.

Don't try to control the uncontrollable.

Many sources of stress are unavoidable and not within control. In an attempt to control the uncontrollable pressure is developed. It may be somehow difficult, but accepting such sources can help you at a later stage.

Forgiveness

We are a combination of right and wrong; no one is perfect. Try to forgive others for their mistakes; give an opportunity. Many times forgiveness also helps to develop a bond. Make yourself free from negative energy by forgiving and move on. Also, remember, you are not for all, and you can't get comfort from all.

Bottom line

Again stress is inevitable in everyone's life. And it is how we respond to our stress stimulus rather than how we react, how we can convert our stress to positive challenges. That can be an opportunity to develop your personality to a rock-solid level. Don't seek pity from others for your stressful situation. You will see many people convert their negative stress to positive challenges, which lead them to success. It is important to understand that stress allows us to grow and develop our personalities.

You are the creator of your destiny. No one can be the expert of your life except you. You may take opinions from others, but it is you who will decide what to do. Blaming others is only the way to a roadblock, blocking your soul, your ideas. You will decide on what you need to give importance to and on what you need not. You will decide what you are going to achieve in your life.

Physical activities like exercise, mediation, yoga, tai-chi, etc., help reduce your day-to-day stress level and build positivity.

And if you are feeling too stressed in life, don't neglect to consult with a professional.

CHAPTER 12

Why Exercise? Way to include exercise in daily routine

The practice of exercise doesn't only improve your physical appearance; exercise helps some more vital ways. Exercise is another keystone habit, performing that also helps in other areas of wellbeing. Everybody knows that exercise is good for health, but we still struggle to do some exercise. Here I am not talking about spending hours in the gym. I am talking about how doing some exercises and being physically active can contribute to wellbeing both mentally and physically. We also talk about how we can incorporate physical activities into our busy lives.

Exercise helps for hormonal balance

Dopamine, serotonin, and norepinephrine, these three major hormones of the monoamine system, are closely connected to your brain activity and emotions. I am making this short. These hormones are responsible for the brain reward system that controls

- Motivation
- Desire, mood
- Feelings of wellbeing
- Cognitive performance
- Stress handling
- Attention, and focusing on performing a task
- Memory storage,
- Sleep, and more.

Low or impaired levels are associated with lack of energy, low concentration, attention deficit, possibly depression, inability to create and act on well-formed plans, or feeling a little down, getting annoyed easily, and more. (1, 2, 3)

All these three major monoamine neurotransmitters, dopamine, norepinephrine, and serotonin, are known to be modulated by exercise. Exercise modulates the direct action of the dopamine system and protects its neuron against toxic assaults. A plethora of evidence from animal and human studies indicates that physical exercise improves health, both physically and mentally. (4, 5)

In a study, researchers from Duke University Medical Center had studied the effect of exercise and medication on people suffering from major depression for 16 weeks. They divided the participants into three groups as

- Exercise group: 3 days of exercise per week, 30 min. each day
- Medication group: Anti-depressant
- And both exercise and medicine.

After four months, patients in all three groups exhibited significant improvement, but the exercise group had shown the biggest improvement. (6)

Regular physical exercise has been proved to have therapeutic benefits such as improved mental health, cognition, and brain function, relieve anxiety, protect the brain against uncontrollable stress, support recovery from brain injury, and resist neurodegenerative diseases like Parkinson's disease and Alzheimer's disease. (7, 8)

According to the Alzheimer's Research & Prevention Foundation, regular physical exercise can drop the risk of developing Alzheimer's disease by up to 50 percent. (9)

Apart from exercise, you can boost norepinephrine and serotonin naturally for better mood through (3)

- Sleep
- Small accomplishments
- Music
- Meditation

- And also eating dopamine rich foods (I don't prefer this much).

Moreover, exercise facilitates weight control, partly through effects on appetite regulation. A review paper of various studies published in the journal of Nutrients suggests that physically active individuals appear to have an improved appetite regulation and may have a closer balance of energy intake and energy expenditure over the longer term. (10) Improper regulation of energy balance, i.e., energy intake and energy expenditure, leads to weight gain.

Does exercise help in sleep?

We have talked about some wellbeing aspects of exercise. This book is for better sleep. Do we have evidence of improvement of sleep by doing exercise? To find it, researchers the National Sleep Foundation's 2013 "Sleep in America" poll studied the sleep habits of 1,000 participants. They found that an overwhelming majority of around 83% of people who exercised at any time of day (including evening<4 h before bed), reported having a better sleep than those who didn't exercise at all. More than 50 percent of vigorous and moderate exercisers slept better on the days when they worked out than on days when they skipped exercise completely. And only 3% who did exercises in the latter part of the night reported worse sleep on days when they exercised, compared to days when they didn't. (11, 12) If you are struggling with sleep, exercise is worth to try.

However, who did vigorous exercise less than one hour before bedtime took a longer time to fall asleep and had poorer sleep quality. (13, 14)

Overall, exercise is one such tool that helps to cope with stress and improve mood, sleep better, and give a better direction towards life.

However, the problem is that the experience of stress also impairs efforts to be physically active. (15)

So, what can we do? Before feeling of stress makes you paralyzed, you need to do exercise to drain stress out. Morning exercise helps to build positivity for the rest of the day.

Not only that, a groundbreaking study conducted by researchers in Belgium, published in the journal of Physiology, suggests that working out early in the morning before breakfast helps to speed up weight loss and boost energy by priming the body for the day. (16)

However, listen to your body, don't go extreme.

How much exercise do you need to perform, and what type?

For most healthy adults, the Department of Health and Human Services recommends these exercise guidelines: (17)

- **Aerobic activity.** Get at least 150 minutes of moderate aerobic activity or 75 minutes of vigorous aerobic activity a week, or a combination of moderate and vigorous activity.
- **Strength training.** Do strength training exercises for all major muscle groups at least two times a week. Aim to do a single set of each exercise, using a weight or resistance level heavy enough to tire your muscles after about 12 to 15 repetitions.

You can break up the whole duration throughout the week at your convenience. For example, if you have work-related stress, do some exercise in the morning time. That can help you to cope with stress and stay positive feelings. Most importantly, you need to enjoy your workout. I prefer to include all types of exercises throughout the week. For example, my workout regime is like two-three days for yoga for core muscles, two days for strength, and two-three days for a short burst (I prefer to do 12 minutes freehand nitric oxide dump exercise) or moderate-intensity exercise in a week. Yoga can be combined with other exercises and for mind-body development. However, I don't have any strict schedule and also miss my day of workout in a week due to my workload. That is not a good thing. I try to include a variety to target different muscles. That also breaks the monotony of exercise, makes it more enjoyable.

If you are a beginner, you may find some difficulty or also may not. Usually, such problems go after 7-10 days.

Including strength training is also necessary. Some people are more inclined to strength to build muscles, and some avoid entirely. Strength training produces different exercise adaptations compared with aerobic exercise and can also be used. (18) The American Heart Association also recommends strength training at least twice per week. (19)

Should older people go for strength training?

Some older people avoid strength training. Research has demonstrated that regular strength-training exercises (e.g., 2 to 3 days per week) help to build muscle strength and muscle mass and preserve bone density, independence, and vitality with age. (20, 21)

As per the Centers for Disease Control and Prevention, Strength training can also reduce the signs and symptoms of many diseases and chronic conditions in older people: (22)

- Arthritis—Reduces pain and stiffness and increases strength and flexibility.
- Diabetes—Improves glycemic control.
- Osteoporosis—Builds bone density and reduces the risk of falls.
- Heart disease—Reduces cardiovascular risk by improving lipid profile and overall fitness. Obesity—Increases metabolism, which helps burn more calories and helps with long-term weight control.
- Back pain—Strengthens back and abdominal muscles to reduce stress on the spine.

The squat is an excellent exercise, whether you are doing with extra weight or not.

If you are new to exercise, it is necessary to evaluate your health status with a healthcare provider's help. Consult with a coach, select some activities to target most parts of the body enjoyably, and carry the same. You can also choose different exercises to get similar results that you can change with your presents to change monotone. You can either join a gym or start in your own home with some small modern equipment or go out to a play area. You will different types of small modern equipment either in a good store or online. Working with a partner makes exercise more enjoyable.

Almost any type of exercise will help. It is always better to do some exercise than do nothing. Most importantly, to continue for the long term, you need to enjoy your workouts. So, make a plan wisely. Another problem I have seen some people spend some time in the gym and sit for rest the whole day. That's not a good habit. Being active is a lifestyle habit.

Tips for doing more exercise

Some easy ways to add more exercise into your daily routine

At the workplace

- Use stairs and find the opportunity to move your body. Stair climbing is very good to burn calories and being active. Downstairs is hard on the knees, so avoid downstairs.
- Move your body at 60 min to 90 min intervals, have a walk inside your workplace, have few minutes talks with someone. Use your phone to set the alarm not to forget. Go for a walk at lunch, tea, or coffee break. Go for a walk at lunch, tea, or coffee break.
- You can do some stretching exercises at your office place; there are many forms of exercise to do at the workplace. Search for some and choose the best suited.
- If you have a question with co-workers, walk to them rather than calling over the phone or sending emails. That will help to move your body along with the clarity of the question. Attend calls in a standing position rather than sitting and can move your body while attending calls.
- Chewing gum: If you are feeling stressed, worked for long hours, try chewing gum, and move your body. Studies found that people who used chewing gum had a lower level of stress. (23, 24) Moderate exercises like walking, also do so. Choose good quality sugarless or low sugar chewing gum.

At the outside

- Walk to your destination as far as possible
- Park your car at a distance so that you can have some walks.

- Take the stairs and skip escalators and elevators at the shopping complex.
- Schedule weekend for fun and activity

At home

- Switch on your favorite music and do some activities that you can enjoy.
- Also, play your music and clean your home.
- Play with or walk your pets.
- Spend some time with your garden. You can build a small garden even if you have less space. Just search for how to build a garden at your home.

Don't be mechanical; don't be obsessed or panic; start with small let it flow gradually, naturally for a sustainable habit. And always listen to your body. Such activities do help not only improving your health but also help to build positivity.

CHAPTER 13

Strategy for wellbeing in life

Our mental health is intimately related to physical health. You may probably feel somewhere in life how hard to achieve physical health with an unhappy mind. You can't achieve sustainable physical health without mental wellbeing. According to a recent June 2020 report from the Journal of American Medical Association-No scientific doubt exists that, mostly, circumstances outside health care nurture or impair health. (1)

Every people mostly realize one day what life is. It matters whether you realize it today or tomorrow. It really matters to understand who you are and what your vision is in life. Be calm, take few minutes deep breath, taking your whole life perspective, imagine what you are going to achieve in your life, what is your identity, will you really be happy with that, how can you climb to that, what is your direction.

It is essential to understand what is important in life and what is not. What can contribute to our mental wellbeing, happiness? What can be the core value of a person? Without understanding the core value, our minds remain confused. If our mind is confused about what to do, we are likely to trap everywhere and likely to move only here and there if we have no direction. We are living globally; we are watching other people and their lifestyle everywhere and trying to follow them. Such behavior mostly builds up our inner dissatisfaction. I am not going to tell you that we should not take a good example of other people. There is a lot to learn from a life of successful people. My point is that those people mostly reach their success in different ways, which may not be relevant for us. If we only watch their lifestyle and wealth, it contributes to our inner dissatisfaction only. We need to adopt what is relevant to our core values.

We will talk about strategies that we can adopt for wellbeing here. I am making it as short as possible. Up to many years of my life, I had no idea about what gives us happiness and contributes to our wellbeing. I was in a confused state of mind, which had a very bad impact on my life, from emotional to physical. I have learned many things from my own life struggles, readings, and other peoples. And I learned many things from Laurie Santos, Cognitive Scientist, and Professor of Psychology at Yale University.

.

External circumstances and happiness

Many people (not all) may think a good income, wealth, luxurious car, home, or buying awesome stuff can make us happy. Your financial position is also a part of your well-being. But if we run blindly after money to buy awesome stuff, we will probably not be happy. A beautiful home can contribute to peace to the mind; however, I am not talking about that point. Joy from external factors like luxurious cars, incentives, buying awesome stuff only contributes a little. After achieving there, that temporary joy declines quickly within a short period. Rather thinking of achieving can give some amount of happiness. Hedonic adaptation is the common tendency of humans to quickly return to a relatively stable state of happiness despite major recent positive or negative events.

For example, if we think a luxurious car can make us happy after years of running, the car's maintenance can make the most common people unhappy. Car is a necessity for many of us-I am not talking that point. What I am talking about is the way of happiness. If someone of our neighbor buys a low-cost car, then we, the luxurious car owner, may have some joy due to our egoistic behavior. But if our neighbor buys a more expensive car, then our egoistic behavior makes us feel more unhappy. I am not going to say that you don't need such stuffs. Rather, I will say concentrating on extra stuff doesn't make us happy as we think. Rather extra stuff makes people frustrated and unhappy- a study from researchers of the University of Illinois at Urbana-Champaign, USA warned (2). You will see some billionaires, super successful people also got depressed. So, external circumstances don't make us as happy as we think commonly. Happiness is more like an inner feeling.

So, what can contribute to long term happiness?

You will see, within the same kind of work, some people enjoy their work, and others don't. Those who find joy in their work, grow in their work type, earn respect and money, and live happily. They can be a good educator, a sports professional, an artist, a renowned guitarist, an environmentalist, a good employee, a nurse, a scientist, or others. You may also call it intrinsic motivation, as they are motivated to repeat the same from their inner character.

This is because their character strength matches up with their work lives. Some people (not all) try to pretend as happy; I am not talking about that. It is an entirely inner feeling. In general, if you are happy on Monday morning to resume your work life, you can consider yourself as happy. Happy people have more freedom. They are more creative and more productive at work.

So, this is a kind of strength of character or a person. These strengths are the positive parts of your personality that impact your thoughts, feelings, and behavior. And this is unique for one. The signature strength of one person may not match with another one. For example, if honesty is your character strength, curiosity is your child, learning or challenging, may be of some others. These are just examples; there are also other types. When someone's character strength is matched us with work-life or professional life, they can find happiness and growth in life. It is the core value of a person. Ignorance of the core value of a happy life is nearly impossible.

Use your signature strength for happiness and growth

You also may see that some people usually stay as happy, which is genetic and can vary from person to person. According to the research model from Professor Sonja Lyubomirsky ((Professor in the Department of Psychology at the University of California, Riverside and author of the bestseller The How of Happiness: A Scientific Approach to Getting the Life You Want)) and colleagues- External life circumstances and a situation like awesome stuff, horrible things have around 10% contribution to happiness or sorrow in life. Apart from genetics, which is 50%, our intention and efforts have about 40% contributions to happiness within our control. (3,4)

Here we have no control over genetics (we can dwarf genetic risks by lifestyle and food choices -I am not talking that), have little control over external circumstance for happiness. But we have control over a significant 40% of our happiness that we can do for a happy life.

Factors Influencing Chronic Happiness Levels

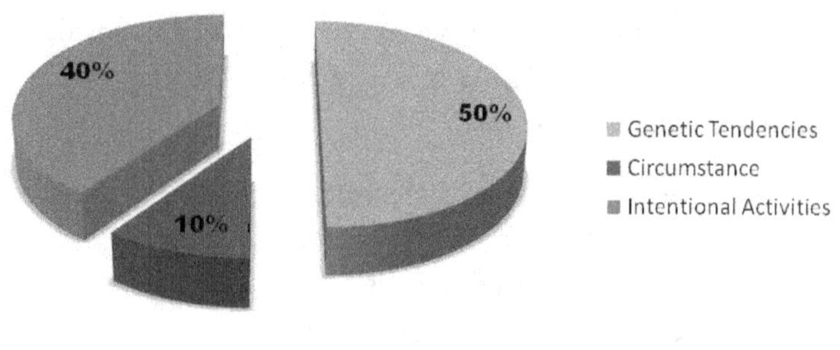

Adapted from Sonja Lyubomirsky's "Pursuing Happiness: The Architecture of Sustainable Change"

Source: Based on Fig. 1 from Review of General Psychology, 2005, Vol. 9, No. 2, 111–131 https://en.wikipedia.org/wiki/Sonja_Lyubomirsky

"Our intentional, effortful activities have a powerful effect on how happy we are, over and above the effects of our set points and the circumstances in which we find ourselves"-Professor Sonja Lyubomirsky (5). Why am I writing on the signature strength?

To continue the practice for intentional and effortful activities, you need to enjoy your activities. Only then can you carry for the long term.

Knowing your character's strength, you will know what type of work can give you happiness. And your right action plan can help you to find a better path for happiness and growth. When the character strength matches up with the career, it can help to flourish your life. You needn't run after money; instead, let money run after you.

It will be incomplete in talking about happiness if we don't talk about the love-affair relationship. True love is unconditional. In love affair relationships, happiness remained at a higher level, and after adapting to marriage, it had come to the normal level after a few years. In a paper published in the Journal of Personality and Social Psychology, researchers from universities such as Michigan State, Brunel University reported. (6)

That means I am not going to tell you not to be married, don't have relationship. We can't deny the importance of a good life partner, a healthy married life, a healthy relationship in our lives. We love people, help others, make other happy-all are good things. Many things, incidents, good or bad, pass through everyone's life. Life is bigger than what comes in and what goes out. Like you can make happy someone, someone can also make you happy. It is also a hard truth that we are all alone at some point in our lives' journey. At some point, happiness is our own. If our happiness lies in someone's hand permanently, it is hard to achieve happiness. We have to do something of our own, which can make us happy apart from our relationships, love for other peoples.

So, I am writing this because knowing your path of happiness, you can do some activities that can give you happiness. Which is important even you are in modern stressful life.

How to know your signature strength of characters

The VIA Institute on Character is a non-profit organization that identifies 24 different character strengths. Although everyone possesses all the characters, the strengths vary in different degrees. That makes each person unique in their character strength profile. The characters with the highest strength are the signature strength of a person.

They have made a tool to identify a person's character strength with multiple-choice questionnaires. You can find out your character strength by answering those questions. You need to be honest while answering the questions to get accurate results. Up to this, VIA Institute provides free information, and you need to register with an email id. You can check your signature strength through VIA research through https://www.viacharacter.org/survey/account/register. Or you can directly online search for 24 character strengths of VIA Institute on Character. I am not affiliated or endorsed with VIA Institute on Character.

How to use your signature strengths in your life

If you need your action plan, you can have it by paying some amount of money to VIA Institute on Character. I have not affiliated with the VIA Institute on Character-for your information. I will not receive any amount of money from the VIA Institute for this. I am not promoting anything; I am just sharing information. If anyone finds it as helpful, it will be my success.

Alternatively, there is another way to have some ideas about the action plan. You can go to my site with this link https://www.holistichealthnlife.com/find-signature-strengths-scientifically-for-growth-happiness/

There you can get a pdf version and can download at free of cost to date.

Goal setting-what goal do you have?

You may have seen many people set goals in a new year to something goods for the year or to overcome a bad habit like cigarette smoking or similar. In my life, I saw most of such goals as a failure.

What may happen if you don't have any goal?

Small or big, goal setting is very important for positive behavior. If you don't have any goal, you don't have a purpose. As we talked earlier, we will just move like here and there mindlessly, watching other people and their lifestyle, feeling unsatisfied or depressed, and likely to be trapped in unhealthy behavior.

You need to be specific about your goal

Someone who just thinks about a goal and takes a few steps without any plan has the very least chance of success in most.

If you have a goal, you will have a clear vision and are less likely to be trapped in unhealthy behavior. To be successful in your goal, you need to very specific about your goal. Again, I like to tell you that **your goal needs to come from your top priorities from the present situation aligned with your vision or future plan, not just watching other people's lifestyles.** Only you can know what your top priority is. You may consult or take advice from your family member who is closely attached to you or professionals, but you are the expert of your life. No one can be the expert of your life; no one knows about your top priority better than you. You need to have a clear vision of what may go to happen, what you will gain and what you will lose, and why. And the ultimate decision of your goal needs to come from you only. Only you can know better what can make you happy. Your wish can be a long-term goal or to perform tomorrow's task. Take a deep breath and release slowly, feel every part of your body, aware of your body, aware of your soul, and imagine what your goal needs to be.

Visualize your goal

While setting a goal, answering questions like what, who, when, how are very important. The goal needs to be quantitative and have a task strategy, like if your goal is four days of exercise in a week, it will be like that on which days, on what time, what types of exercise, and how long you will do exercise. Your goal can be to build a habit of doing exercise five days a week, complete a task in ten days, or long terms like changing your carrier or better health. You need to break the long-term goal into shorter time-bound short goals.

And remember, your goal needs to be meaningful, feasible but also needs to be a little bit difficult. For example, in the long term, seven days of exercise in a week can be very hard for a common person; starting from three days a week to make a habit of five days of exercise in a week is achievable.

Your goal needs to be:

- Specific needs to come from your top priorities from the present situation aligned with your vision or future plan of your life
- Measurable-outcome of your need to be measured, like whether some change in life for the better, achieving something, completion of a task or like that
- Time bound-when you are going to start your goal and when you are going to complete
- Realistic- You definitely need to have a realistic goal.
- A little bit hard but achievable for you. A very easy goal often leads to boredom, and unrealistic goal may lead to frustration

How many goals at a time?

Choosing too many goals at a time often leads to failure. That will be like moving here and there rather than moving towards the goal. Choosing one or two goals at a time will be better. Or if the goals are the smaller ones, you may stretch to one more. If you have a big goal, work on it, break it down into small goals. Everything needs to be noted. If you note it, your brain will be released, and you are unlikely to forget some of the important tasks over time.

Once you have identified your goal, it is time to visualize your goal. It is like what will happen if you achieve the goal, how it will feel when you achieve it, or what else you don't like.

You need to visualize the obstacles, your strength, recourses, and weakness during goal visualization. This is what we call mental contrasting. In a two-year follow-up study, researchers from Columbia University found that women who learned mental contrast had succeeded in goals better than those who hadn't. (10) You need to be alone, calm, and uninterrupted for a few minutes for the whole goal-setting process.

You need to look at your past experience, your mistakes, and your success. It is crucial to find out the obstacles and take them to the deep. You may have obstacles from your own inside and from the outside environment. Mostly the inner obstacles are more significant than the external constraints that we understand very little. We are the biggest enemy of ourselves. Most of the time, our negative thoughts, emotions, excuses, our own beliefs, our mindset (like a fixed mindset that we can grow), our bad habits, our ego are the biggest enemies of our own. If such behavior is at the top of our lives, we don't need any other enemy to ruin our lives.

Horrible things happen in everyone's life. It depends on how you respond to them. When you overcome your inner impediments, you can find a path. Remember, without finding out the obstacle; your behavior will be empty.

Gabriele Oettingen, professor of psychology, draws on more than twenty years of research in the Science of human motivation to reveal why conventional wisdom falls short. (11)

To achieve the goal, you need to think and act in a very specific way

You have shorted out your Strength, weakness, and recourses, identified for your goal. Now time to plan and organize your activities.

- Identify your goal with measurable-outcome, your need to be measured, like whether some change in life for the better, completion of a task within a specified time.
- Visualization, Analysis resources, Strength, and weakness, ask yourself what you can do to overcome your weakness if necessary, take help from an expert. You may also need to adjust yourself somewhere in your life. You will not get all the fruits at the same time. You may need to leave some to have the better one.
- Time Factor: how much time you are going to for your goal. Time to start, time to complete, and

- Planning and organizing activities, if required, you need to outsource less important activities so that you can focus on the core part of your goal.
- Put it into action
- Review the progress at the interval: You need to review your plan timely. Many things change with time, and you may need some adjustment with your action plan over time. And you need to note down all your plan, failure, obstacles, and progress. It is better to review at the weekend and plan for the next week.
- Re-adjust, re-organize activities, if there is any need of that
- Put it into action

To achieve our goal, we need to pass through different stages; we may need support from outside or sometimes from a professional who may be an expert on some work that you may need. One common mistake is that we often go to master everything. But the truth is we can't be masters on everything. We may sometimes need help from professionals. Your main focus will be on your goal's core area and other related supportive action you may require from outside resources.

And nothing will happen unless and until you are not taking any step of your plan towards your goal. For a long-term goal, your continuous effort will be needed. A tree will not give you fruits on the next day; you need to take care of it.

Cus D'Amato and Mike Tyson

You may probably hear about Mike Tyson, one of the ferocious boxing champions, stepped inside the ring, and who had become the youngest heavyweight boxing champion of the world at the age of 20. But a hidden side of him very fewer people know about his success was his coach Constantine D'Amato who had handled the carrier of Mike Tyson. In his childhood, Mike Tyson lived in society's crust, surrounded by criminals, poverty, and crime. Tyson was repeatedly caught committing petty crimes and fighting those who ridiculed his high-pitched voice and lisp. Constantine D'Amato had given Mike Tyson a very important life lesson. He trained Tyson not to fight with people, not to fight with his ego but fight to win fights. D'Amato reinforced his mentality over and over, trained him to convert his violent attitude, behavioral and emotional problems to win fights, and the result was the youngest world heavyweight boxing champion. (7,8,9)

Self-evaluation of your time spend

Time is one big valuable in everyone's life. Somewhere I read (I apologize that I cannot remember right now), "*if you value your time, others will value you, and if you don't value your time, you need to depend on others.*"

It would be best if you give value to your time. We often say that we have no time to do something new. Time is our own. The way how we spend our time, the return will also in the same way.

Recently I went through a person telling me like life has nothing, let's have a drink. I asked why you are telling like that. The reply was like that in office he had to follow his boss's order, in the home he had the burden of family and close ones. I asked how much time in a day you were giving for yourself. After some moments of silence, he replied he was actually not giving any time for himself. He admitted that he had spent not less than two hours mindless scrolling cell phone and television channels after going through his daily schedule. I asked again can your cut some of those time and spend it on your own or something peaceful or creative. The reply was positive.

If we are not giving any time for our wellbeing, how can we aspect a happy life? Even you are dedicated to spending your life to help others; you need to give some time for your wellbeing to carry your dedication.

You may hear in attending fight telling to wear your mask at first before helping others in the case of emergency.

Mindless scrolling of social media, television channels, spending hour to hour to find a dress, watching other people's wealth or lifestyle, watching porn are definitely not the time we are spending for ours. I am not going to tell you that you don't watch social media or television channels. Rather I am going to tell you to be mindful, specific rather than mindless scrolling. Everything has its own positive and negative sides, and it depends on the end person who picks it.

Before telling that we have no time, it is essential to know how we are spending our time.

Evaluate what type of activities you are spending your time and note it down. Check whether you can adjust your time to do something positive. For example, see whether you can cut some time from keeping the smart-phone away and do some exercise or something good for your goal.

Mind Control

Here it means controlling our own mind, not other peoples. Our mind doesn't only fix at a point; it flows over other things. And minds are not staying with us most of the time. Mind-wandering is the experience of thoughts not remaining on a single topic for a long period, particularly when people are engaged in an attention-demanding task. (13)

It is like you are trying to complete a task and you are thinking about whether you will go shopping or not. This is a widespread problem. If you have a goal, you need to focus on it. Your time is valuable.

In different parts of our brain, do a particular task, focus on different things. The default network of the brain becomes active when you are not involved in a task. This network of your brain can take your mind from the present job to somewhere else within a second. And your mind can go to the future or past from the present moment within a second. And you stop doing your task.

In a study from Harvard University, Cambridge, Matthew A. Killingsworth,And Daniel T. Gilbert found people mind-wander 46.9% of the time, and mind-wandering makes us feel bad. (14)

Exercise-Meditation to stop Mind-wandering

If your mind is racing, you cannot focus due to distracting thoughts; meditation is worth trying. Practicing meditation helps to turn the mind away from distracting thoughts to a single point. A study from a research team from Yale University found meditation stops mind-wandering. They found the default network is less active, and other brain regions are more active in meditators than other control peoples. (15)

If adverse environments surround you, meditation is a handy tool to bring a positive feeling. Meditation not only helps to calm and improve attention during the meditation time, but it also enhances its wellness to the later stage. A few minutes of meditation helps in many ways: (16)

- Reduce stress
- Control anxiety
- Promote emotional health
- Enhance self-awareness
- Helps to be present in the moments, lengthen attention span
- May fight addictions
- Can generate kindness
- Improves sleep and more

The 4-7-8 breath is also known as the Relaxing Breath. This technique is used to calm down your mind and achieve a desired mental or physical state. It is effortless, requires no room, and can be done nearly in no time. It involves deep breathing in for 4 seconds, holding the breath for 7 seconds, and exhaling for 8 seconds.

Step 1: Sit comfortably and keep your back straight. Keep your lips slightly apart and exhale completely through your mouth, making a whooshing sound.

Step 2: Close your lips and inhale quietly through your nose. Count for four seconds in the mind while inhaling

Step 3: Hold your breath for a count of seven seconds in mind.

Step 4: Exhale completely through your mouth, with a whoosh sound for eight seconds.

This completes one cycle. Try for another three cycles. Note that start with exhale audibly through your mouth and inhale quietly through your nose and. And don't be too alert. Feel your spinal cord, stomach, the whole body during the process. You may not achieve in a single day; some practices make it perfect.

You can learn more with 4-7-8 Breath from Dr. Andrew Weil's video. You can find by searching in search engine like Google.

There are different types of meditation. Even a few minutes of deep breathing helps to control the mind. Investing 5-10 min in meditation is a healthy practice in a positive direction. If your mind is racing and you are not able to sleep, meditation is worth a try. You can find a different way of meditation. Juts need to feel your body, your forehead, face, neck, spinal cord, stomach, feet etc, aware your soul. Practice makes it perfect. A small three to four-minute light exercise also helps to keep away from other distractions and focus on work.

Frequent watching of the cell phone is another reason for shifting our minds. You can keep your phone away during work time or keep in a place where you have to put some effort to reach the phone. You can shape your environment less bad as possible.

Social connection, family, friend, pet

Humans are social animals. No amount of education, money, privilege, or success can safeguard you against disconnection and loneliness. Can you imagine a situation of living alone on an Island? How long we can survive in such a case, even we have a high level of fitness, foods to eat, and strong willpower. Probably many of us can't survive for a long time. I am not about the Jungle Book story where Mowgli had adopted the jungle's life with animals' friendship from childhood. I am talking about if one of us had to live on a lonely island without connecting with others. Probably we can't. That's why we need society even we have foods to eat and are mentally and physically strong. Social connection enhances the richness of life, boosts mood, and keeps you away from loneliness.

But, although we are connected with many people in traditional social media, we haven't reduced our feelings of disconnect and loneliness many times.

Many of these are per-formative interactions rather than meaningful, human conversations: "I like your post" vs. "I understand something about you and want you to understand me, too." Such kind of interaction is not going to help much. On the positive side, technology creates new opportunities to connect with others and can offer a bridge to those who struggle to make in-person contact. But the capacity for negative impact exists, too; social media can cause real pain and alienation when trolling, bullying, ghosting, popularity contests, and images of perfection (reinforcing the insecurity that "you are not enough") are prevalent.-explained Lara Otte, Psy.D., The Human Connection in Psychology Today. (17)

But there are other opportunities with social media. We have the opportunity to have a world-wide connection, can have a circle of like-minded people, share ideas, can express the feeling of joy. If you are not finding social support from your physical surrounding, you can find a good community of your own kind. You can also find your missing friend. Social media also gives the opportunity to learn more. It depends on how you use social media. Binge-watching is obviously not the right choice. Moreover, using social media in the right way can give you the excellent potential to inspire and connect people.

We need some meaningful conversation to safeguard our loneliness in the real world. Apart from your family member, you can have a good social circle from your surrounding; friends have some friendly talks, joy at least once a week, if not daily. Or at least have some conversation even over the phone, if your friend is far away from you.

There are also some other ways; we can connect with others. To boost mood, you need not necessarily be connected with your best friend. Even a simple act of talking to a stranger on the street helps to boost moods more than we expect. Researchers found talking to strangers makes us happy. Even if you are reluctant to talk to a stranger, you and the stranger get a happiness boost after meaningful talking to each other. (18)

In another study, researchers found sharing something good with others makes them better. (19) For example, you can share your delicious food with other people and feel happiness.

There are nothing any hard and fast rules. Social connection can be an eye connection, a smile, a simple talk, or similar. You may imagine how a teen feels with eye contact with the beloved. What can we do? Simply have a small conversation with someone when you go for a walk; when you are traveling in public transports, (rather than spending time with the smart-phone), with someone in the coffee shop or even with the co-workers or like that. It is just like searching for an opportunity to connect with others positively. Having connected socially also helps to overcome traits of introversion.

Tip: Develop a circle of like-minded people who are doing similar things to you and share ideas. A trustworthy digital community can also help you many times. Sometimes adjust your time a little and use public transport.

Having a pet is also good company and helps to relieve your stress. Friendship with a pet is a divine relation. A pet doesn't judge you; they can return pure love. A study also found that the loneliest individuals benefited from visits with dogs. (20)

Art is another thing that can help to relieve stress, even though you may not be good at art. You can take part in your child's artwork. That also helps to improve your bindings with your child with quality time.

Savoring, Gratitude, Kindness

Savoring is the way by which we attempt to fully feel, enjoy, and extend our positive experiences. It is a great way to develop a long-lasting stream of positive experiences and emotions. It involves stepping outside of an experience that you feel good to review and appreciate.

For example, you visited a beautiful park, watched a good movie, read a good book, had a pleasant walk, enrolled in a great course, or something similar that can give you a feel-good experience. And share your experience with another person. That also keeps your attention, and you will be absorbed by the moment. Note down what makes you happy and use your phone to take a picture to realize it later. That also helps to lengthen your positive emotion.

Express gratitude, show appreciation. Taking time to experience gratitude can make you happier and even healthier. You can note down the things that make you grateful, happy, taking 5-10 minutes at night. That can help you to explore more, and plan accordingly.

You may consider kindness as a simple act of doing something nice. Doing nice stuff like helping others, needy, giving food to the hungry, volunteering to a community, help to improve your mood. You needn't necessarily do something big to be kind.

These are small things that we can perform without a big cost.

Laughing, cuddling, hugging, kissing, having sex

Laughter is good therapy to relieve stress and relaxing tension in muscles. Small things, activities like cuddling, hugging, kissing, and having sex can help enjoy better mental health, quality of life, and lower stress. (21, 22) Even self-hugging can be beneficial.

Doing nothing sometimes, staying with Nature

As a child, I was told a story of a sleepless king. A very busy king was unable to sleep at night. After many experts failed, the king announced a reward to anyone who could make him sleep. And a little girl came forward to the king. The girl brought the king under the open sky that night. The king had forgotten to feel Nature during his busy schedule and felt very relaxed while looking at the sky, the twinkling stars, and soon fell asleep there.

In the present busy environment, many of us even forget ourselves.

If you are exhausted with the workload, tired with a racing mind or clogged thoughts, then find some time on your own. Stay sometimes with Nature and doing nothing can help to bring peace to your brain. Many times, doing nothing or an empty account in a hectic life is very relaxing. That also helps to rethink the unthinkable.

The power and beauty of Nature can bring us immediately to the present moment, keeping aside the other things that are also a way of mindfulness. You can watch how a bird is flying, how a cloud is moving, how a star is twinkling, or similar.

For example, a study found that looking at trees and Nature's photos helped people recover from stressful encounters. (23) In a review, researchers from several universities like the University of Washington, Stanford University, University of Chicago, Wageningen University and Research, University of Bristol, and more, suggest keeping touch with Nature for mental wellbeing. (24)

What can we do? We can create a small garden if we have some space. Sitting in a park or resort also gives a nature-like feeling, peace of mind. You can plan your weekend in such a place. If you live in a stressful life and plan for a holiday trip, don't involve too many activities. Just participate in a few events, relax and enjoy the journey.

Having sunlight exposure in a controlled manner

In our busy lives, we mostly forget about sunlight. Our ancestors were regularly exposed to sunlight. That also helps to keep many diseases away. Daylight is another key in regulating daily sleep patterns. NIH recommends being outside in natural sunlight for at least 30 minutes each day. (25)

That will also help you to get vitamin D. MoreoverVitamin D plays many roles inside your body, including promoting serotonin production. And therefore having sunlight also helps to boost mood by boosting serotonin production that controls our mood. (26)

I was once asked by one of my friends –I have a very less open place in my apartment, how can I have sunlight? It is very simple. Take a chair to the balcony with a book or some of the daily activities that you can do while sitting. If you don't have a balcony, open a window, and sit there. It is just an idea of how you can implement it in your life.

However, consult with your doctor before having sunlight as you may have skin disorders or sensitivity.

Take some pain

There is a word, no pain, no gain. Easy coming goes easy. Taking some pain to do some hard target many times turns things to a better side. Again, that needs to be reasonable and achievable in your life. Taking pain to do a hard goal helps to break out from the comfort zone. It would be best if you found out the edge of your comfort zone. If we spend most of our time in the comfort zone, many goals are not feasible, and stress begins to develop. Only those win who has the right goal strategy, execute and never surrender. Excuses are a way to failure. Telling your sad story, seeking pity, many times kills our willpower. To fulfill your dream, you have to do it your own. I am not talking about teamwork to complete a task. I am talking about our personal goals. At some point in life, we all are alone-this is the truth of life. We have to assess our resources to achieve a goal. Without a goal, a dream is only a dream. Embrace the hurdles, the sadness. Most successful people learn from their mistakes and never give up—all you need courage and resolution to take some pain and do things. And if you find it hard to deal with some of your hurdles in your life, it is worthy to consult with a professional.

If you are seeking a permanent solution to your condition like ill health, financial or job-related problems, you need a solid plan. Ill-health contributes to unhappiness. You need to find the right healthcare provider, health, and life coach to evaluate your health and make a solid plan. If something is hindering you from achieving your goal, from coming out from your condition, you can try Julie Morgenstern's SHED-A Four-Step Guide to Getting Unstuck.

"I don't believe that any book (including this book) is a fix-all, magic pill. I won't promise this book will solve your problems, help you find peace, or reveal the secret of life. It won't. What I will promise, however, is that reading this book will dislodge from your current state of paralysis and help you move forward with optimism and confidence."- Julie Morgenstern

A good book often changes your life in a positive direction, which is worth much more than it cost. Again, don't be frustrated with your work or goal. The harder you work, the brighter your results. Many small things that many people don't think about can give a big change. You just need to figure out what will work for you.

FINAL THOUGHTS

We have learned several things about foods and lifestyle strategies. I am not telling you that I follow all those things all the time. But I can tell you that I follow some that suit my life and give me good results. We get results when something fits our lives. Only then we can carry it for a long time.

There is no magic pill in life. However, knowledge is always something special. But we can't just learn the stuff and sit. Learning is not going to give any result unless and until we put it into action. But if we know the reason we can take the step. And things do not happen in a single day. If you want to change something for good, you need at least some amount of intentional effort. It is crucial to evaluate our habits and what needs to change for good-I like to say again. When things go in a better way, it begins to give joy day by day. If you cannot do exercise seven days a week, you are performing four days a week; it is ok. Everyone starts in that way. Like most of us who want to change something in life; sometimes, I also struggled in the beginning.

Once you change something for goods, it becomes like a habit after a few days or weeks. Your subconscious mind then picks it up. It then goes comfortably in life like brushing your teeth in the morning, washing your hair with shampoo, driving to your office, and like that. That is the power of the subconscious mind. So once you can maintain a regular time for bed, a lot of things will be pleased. And it would be best if you found the kinds of stuff which fits your life. Many times after trying different kinds of stuff, you can find a better way. Priority is finding some time, like cutting some time from scrolling in the smart-phone or social media and try to spend that time on something worthy. Also, remember choosing too many activities at a time often leads to failure. It is better to starts with one or two.

And if you are continuously having trouble sleeping, you should consult with your health care provider.

Self-evaluation is one most crucial part. Many time our own beliefs, our own emotions, our bad habits hinder in achieving a goal rather than the external environment-I like to repeat.

Your body is one of your best friends, who is continuously working for you. Your body's first and foremost priority is to keep you alive. If you ignore your body, you are bound to pay. We are bound to give our time to health, whether with a healthy life or sickness. Without a healthy life, with lots of pain in the body, happiness is nearly impossible. And without happiness and well-being, sustainable health is not possible. It is all about happiness, to have joy in life.

And lastly, I like to repeat that to constantly support your mental well-being; you need a like-minded community that needs to have positive thoughts and creative ideas. If you don't have physically around you, at least have in the digital world like social media. Interact positively with others, respect others, share positive thoughts, creative ideas, and have ideas from others, and participate in well-being. But don't watch binge on social media. And always value your time, but don't be mechanical. Life is like a roller coaster. We fall, learn from mistakes. And we rise.

I hope you have enjoyed the book. And most importantly, it will be great if you spend little of your valuable time to leave your honest feedback. I am not very good at writing. If anything I have missed here, it will be a great value for me and other peoples. I wrote this book as a part of my upcoming book on ending sugar craving permanently and losing extra weight. To health and happiness-it is my good wish to you.

.

REFERENCES

Chapter 1: A call from a Friend

1. Teresa Arora, PhD, Sleep Doesn't Waste Time, It's Good for the Waist Line, *Sleep*, Volume 38, Issue 8, August 2015, Pages 1159–1160, https://doi.org/10.5665/sleep.4884

2.Sutanto, C.N.; Wang, M.X.; Tan, D.; Kim, J.E. Association of Sleep Quality and Macronutrient Distribution: A Systematic Review and Meta-Regression. *Nutrients* 2020, *12*, 126.

3. https://www.sleepfoundation.org/articles/what-happens-when-you-sleep

4.Xie L, Kang H, Xu Q, et al. Sleep drives metabolite clearance from the adult brain. *Science*. 2013;342(6156):373-377. doi:10.1126/science.1241224

5.Malkki, H. Sleep alleviates AD-related neuropathological processes. *Nat Rev Neurol* 9, 657 (2013). https://doi.org/10.1038/nrneurol.2013.230

6.Robbins R, Quan SF, Weaver MD, Bormes G, Barger LK, Czeisler CA. Examining sleep deficiency and disturbance and their risk for incident dementia and all-cause mortality in older adults across 5 years in the United States. Aging (Albany NY). 2021 Feb 11;13. doi: 10.18632/aging.202591. Epub ahead of print. PMID: 33570509

7.Coupled electrophysiological, hemodynamic, and cerebrospinal fluid oscillations in human sleep BY NINA E. FULTZ, GIORGIO BONMASSAR, KAWIN SETSOMPOP, ROBERT A. STICKGOLD, BRUCE R. ROSEN, JONATHAN R. POLIMENI, LAURA D. LEWIS SCIENCE01 NOV 2019 : 628-631, DOI: 10.1126/science.aax5440

8.Christoph Nissen, Hannah Piosczyk, Johannes Holz, Jonathan G Maier, Lukas Frase, Annette Sterr, Dieter Riemann, Bernd Feige, Sleep is more than rest for plasticity in the human cortex, *Sleep*, 2021;, zsaa216, https://doi.org/10.1093/sleep/zsaa216

Chapter 2: Sleep deprivation, Food Craving, Weight gain and many health disorders

1.Sutanto, C.N.; Wang, M.X.; Tan, D.; Kim, J.E. Association of Sleep Quality and Macronutrient Distribution: A Systematic Review and Meta-Regression. *Nutrients* **2020**, *12*, 126.

2. van Dalfsen JH, Markus CR. The influence of sleep on human hypothalamic-pituitary-adrenal (HPA) axis reactivity: A systematic review. *Sleep Med Rev.* 2018;39:187–194. doi:10.1016/j.smrv.2017.10.002

3. Vargas I, Lopez-Duran N. Investigating the effect of acute sleep deprivation on hypothalamic-pituitary-adrenal-axis response to a psychosocial stressor. *Psychoneuroendocrinology.* 2017;79:1–8. doi:10.1016/j.psyneuen.2017.01.030

4.https://www.sleepfoundation.org/articles/connection-between-sleep-and-overeating

5.University Of Chicago Medical Center. "Sleep Loss Boosts Appetite, May Encourage Weight Gain." ScienceDaily. ScienceDaily, 7 December 2004. <www.sciencedaily.com/releases/2004/12/041206210355.htm>.

6. Ness KM, Strayer SM, Nahmod NG, et al. Four nights of sleep restriction suppress the postprandial lipemic response and decrease satiety. *J Lipid Res.* 2019;60(11):1935–1945. doi:10.1194/jlr.P094375

7.St-Onge, Marie-Pierre et al. "Effects of Diet on Sleep Quality." *Advances in nutrition (Bethesda, Md.)* vol. 7,5 938-49. 15 Sep. 2016, doi:10.3945/an.116.012336

8.Zuraikat FM, Makarem N, Liao M, St-Onge MP, Aggarwal B. Measures of Poor Sleep Quality Are Associated With Higher Energy Intake and Poor Diet Quality in a Diverse Sample of Women From the Go Red for Women Strategically Focused Research Network. *J Am Heart Assoc.* 2020;9(4):e014587. doi:10.1161/JAHA.119.014587

9. Greer SM, Goldstein AN, Walker MP. The impact of sleep deprivation on food desire in the human brain. *Nat Commun.* 2013;4:2259. doi:10.1038/ncomms3259

10.Rihm JS, Menz MM, Schultz H, et al. Sleep Deprivation Selectively Upregulates an Amygdala-Hypothalamic Circuit Involved in Food Reward. *J Neurosci*. 2019;39(5):888–899. doi:10.1523/JNEUROSCI.0250-18.2018

11. Beebe DW, Simon S, Summer S, Hemmer S, Strotman D, Dolan LM. Dietary intake following experimentally restricted sleep in adolescents. *Sleep*. 2013;36(6):827–834. Published 2013 Jun 1. doi:10.5665/sleep.2704

12. Simon SL, Field J, Miller LE, DiFrancesco M, Beebe DW. Sweet/dessert foods are more appealing to adolescents after sleep restriction. *PLoS One*. 2015;10(2):e0115434. Published 2015 Feb 23. doi:10.1371/journal.pone.0115434

13. St-Onge MP, Wolfe S, Sy M, Shechter A, Hirsch J. Sleep restriction increases the neuronal response to unhealthy food in normal-weight individuals. *Int J Obes (Lond)*. 2014;38(3):411–416. doi:10.1038/ijo.2013.114

14. St-Onge MP, McReynolds A, Trivedi ZB, Roberts AL, Sy M, Hirsch J. Sleep restriction leads to increased activation of brain regions sensitive to food stimuli. *Am J Clin Nutr*. 2012;95(4):818–824. doi:10.3945/ajcn.111.027383

15.Baum KT, Desai A, Field J, Miller LE, Rausch J, Beebe DW. Sleep restriction worsens mood and emotion regulation in adolescents. *J Child Psychol Psychiatry*. 2014;55(2):180–190. doi:10.1111/jcpp.12125

<u>16.</u> Beebe DW, Fallone G, Godiwala N, et al. Feasibility and behavioral effects of an at-home multi-night sleep restriction protocol for adolescents. *J Child Psychol Psychiatry*. 2008;49(9):915–923. doi:10.1111/j.1469-7610.2008.01885.x

17.Lack of Sleep and Diabetes, Written by Danielle Pacheco, Medically Reviewed by Dr. Abhinav Singh, Sleep Foundation, November 20, 2020 https://www.sleepfoundation.org/physical-health/lack-of-sleep-and-diabetes

18. Broussard JL, Ehrmann DA, Van Cauter E, Tasali E, Brady MJ. Impaired insulin signaling in human adipocytes after experimental sleep restriction: a randomized, crossover study. *Ann Intern Med*. 2012;157(8):549–557. doi:10.7326/0003-4819-157-8-201210160-00005

19.Sweeney EL, Jeromson S, Hamilton DL, Brooks NE, Walshe IH. Skeletal muscle insulin signaling and whole-body glucose metabolism following acute sleep restriction in healthy males. *Physiol Rep*. 2017;5(23):e13498. doi:10.14814/phy2.13498

20.Rao MN, Neylan TC, Grunfeld C, Mulligan K, Schambelan M, Schwarz JM. Subchronic sleep restriction causes tissue-specific insulin resistance. *J Clin Endocrinol Metab.* 2015;100(4):1664–1671. doi:10.1210/jc.2014-3911

21. Rao MN, Neylan TC, Grunfeld C, Mulligan K, Schambelan M, Schwarz JM. Subchronic sleep restriction causes tissue-specific insulin resistance. *J Clin Endocrinol Metab.* 2015;100(4):1664–1671. doi:10.1210/jc.2014-3911

22. Cedernaes, J., Lampola, L., Axelsson, E.K., Liethof, L., Hassanzadeh, S., Yeganeh, A., Broman, J.-E., Schiöth, H.B. and Benedict, C. (2016), A single night of partial sleep loss impairs fasting insulin sensitivity but does not affect cephalic phase insulin release in young men. J Sleep Res, 25: 5-10. doi:10.1111/jsr.12340

23. Donga E, van Dijk M, van Dijk JG, et al. A single night of partial sleep deprivation induces insulin resistance in multiple metabolic pathways in healthy subjects. J Clin Endocrinol Metab. 2010;95(6):2963–2968. doi:10.1210/jc.2009-2430

24.Reutrakul S, Hood MM, Crowley SJ, Morgan MK, Teodori M, Knutson KL, Van Cauter E. Chronotype is independently associated with glycemic control in type 2 diabetes. Diabetes Care. 2013 Sep;36(9):2523-9. doi: 10.2337/dc12-2697. Epub 2013 May 1. PMID: 23637357; PMCID: PMC3747872. https://pubmed.ncbi.nlm.nih.gov/23637357/

25.Leproult R, Holmbäck U, Van Cauter E. Circadian misalignment augments markers of insulin resistance and inflammation, independently of sleep loss. Diabetes. 2014 Jun;63(6):1860-9. doi: 10.2337/db13-1546. Epub 2014 Jan 23. PMID: 24458353; PMCID: PMC4030107. https://pubmed.ncbi.nlm.nih.gov/24458353/

26.Broussard JL, Chapotot F, Abraham V, et al. Sleep restriction increases free fatty acids in healthy men. Diabetologia. 2015;58(4):791–798. doi:10.1007/s00125-015-3500-4

27. Nedeltcheva AV, Scheer FA. Metabolic effects of sleep disruption, links to obesity and diabetes. *Curr Opin Endocrinol Diabetes Obes.* 2014;21(4):293–298. doi:10.1097/MED.0000000000000082

28. Reutrakul S, Van Cauter E. Sleep influences on obesity, insulin resistance, and risk of type 2 diabetes. *Metabolism.* 2018;84:56–66. doi:10.1016/j.metabol.2018.02.010

29. Sleeping more on weekends does not make up for past sleep loss,

Written by Maria Cohut, Ph.D. Fact checked by Isabel Godfrey, Medical News Today March 4, 2019, https://www.medicalnewstoday.com/articles/324610

30. Alhola P, Polo-Kantola P. Sleep deprivation: Impact on cognitive performance. *Neuropsychiatr Dis Treat*. 2007;3(5):553–567

31. Killgore WD. Effects of sleep deprivation on cognition. *Prog Brain Res*. 2010;185:105–129. doi:10.1016/B978-0-444-53702-7.00007-5

32. Dai XJ, Jiang J, Zhang Z, et al. Plasticity and Susceptibility of Brain Morphometry Alterations to Insufficient Sleep. *Front Psychiatry*. 2018;9:266. Published 2018 Jun 27. doi:10.3389/fpsyt.2018.00266

33.How Sleep Strengthens Your Immune System, by Elizabeth Pratt, Healthline, February 20, 2019, https://www.healthline.com/health-news/how-sleep-bolsters-your-immune-system

34.Fernandes, P.A., Kinker, G.S., Navarro, B.V., Jardim, V.C., Ribeiro-Paz, E.D., Córdoba-Moreno, M.O., Santos-Silva, D., Muxel, S.M., Fujita, A., Moraes, C., Nakaya, H.I., Buckeridge, M.S. and Markus, R.P. 2021. Melatonin-Index as a biomarker for predicting the distribution of presymptomatic and asymptomatic SARS-CoV-2 carriers. *Melatonin Research*. 4, 1 (Jan. 2021), 189-205. DOI:https://doi.org/https://doi.org/10.32794/mr11250090.

35.How Sleep Affects Immunity, by Eric Suni, reviewed by Dr. Kimberly Truong, SleepFoundation.org, November 19, 2020, https://www.sleepfoundation.org/physical-health/how-sleep-affects-immunity

36.NIOSH Training for Nurses on Shift Work and Long Work Hours, Sleep and the Immune System, Centers for Disease Control and Prevention https://www.cdc.gov/niosh/work-hour-training-for-nurses/longhours/mod2/05.html

37. Zhao Z, Zhao X, Veasey SC. Neural Consequences of Chronic Short Sleep: Reversible or Lasting?. *Front Neurol*. 2017;8:235. Published 2017 May 31. doi:10.3389/fneur.2017.00235

38. Ness KM, Strayer SM, Nahmod NG, Chang AM, Buxton OM, Shearer GC. Two nights of recovery sleep restores the dynamic lipemic response, but not the reduction of insulin sensitivity, induced by five nights of sleep restriction. *Am J Physiol Regul Integr Comp Physiol*. 2019;316(6):R697–R703. doi:10.1152/ajpregu.00336.2018

39. St-Onge, Marie-Pierre et al. "Effects of Diet on Sleep Quality." *Advances in nutrition (Bethesda, Md.)* vol. 7,5 938-49. 15 Sep. 2016, doi:10.3945/an.116.012336

40. https://www.apa.org/monitor/2017/10/cover-sleep

41.https://www.webmd.com/sleep-disorders/features/10-results-sleep-loss#1

42.https://www.nhs.uk/live-well/sleep-and-tiredness/why-lack-of-sleep-is-bad-for-your-health/

43. https://www.mayoclinic.org/healthy-lifestyle/adult-health/expert-answers/how-many-hours-of-sleep-are-enough/faq-20057898

44. Hirshkowitz M, Whiton K, Albert SM, et al. National Sleep Foundation's sleep time duration recommendations: methodology and results summary. *Sleep Health*. 2015;1(1):40–43. doi:10.1016/j.sleh.2014.12.010

Chapter 3: What is the best time for sleep-Circadian Rhythm

1.https://en.wikipedia.org/wiki/Circadian_rhythm

2.https://www.nigms.nih.gov/education/pages/factsheet circadianrhythms.aspx

3. Souza RV, Sarmento RA, de Almeida JC, Canuto R. The effect of shift work on eating habits: a systematic review. *Scand J Work Environ Health*. 2019;45(1):7–21. doi:10.5271/sjweh.3759

4. Gupta CC, Coates AM, Dorrian J, Banks S. The factors influencing the eating behaviour of shiftworkers: what, when, where and why. *Ind Health*. 2019;57(4):419–453. doi:10.2486/indhealth.2018-0147

5. Lopez-Minguez J, Gómez-Abellán P, Garaulet M. Timing of Breakfast, Lunch, and Dinner. Effects on Obesity and Metabolic Risk. *Nutrients*. 2019;11(11):2624. Published 2019 Nov 1. doi:10.3390/nu11112624

6. Okada C, Imano H, Muraki I, Yamada K, Iso H. The Association of Having a Late Dinner or Bedtime Snack and Skipping Breakfast with Overweight in Japanese Women. *J Obes*. 2019;2019:2439571. Published 2019 Mar 3. doi:10.1155/2019/2439571
https://www.ncbi.nlm.nih.gov/pmc/articles/PMC6421799/

7. What Are the Best Hours to Sleep?, National Sleep Foundation, https://www.sleep.org/articles/best-hours-sleep/

8.Earth's Magnetic Field (compass needles), Science On a Sphere®
https://sos.noaa.gov/datasets/earths-magnetic-field-compass-needles/

9.What happens when magnetic north and true north align?, by Paul Wilkes, The Conversation, September 17 2019Science X™
https://phys.org/news/2019-09-magnetic-north-true-align.html

10.What the Principles of Feng Shui and Vastu Shastra Say About Sleep Direction, Medically reviewed by Debra Rose Wilson, Ph.D., MSN, R.N., IBCLC, AHN-BC, CHT — Written by Kristeen Cherney, September 30, 2019, HealthLine https://www.healthline.com/health/best-direction-to-sleep

11.Hekmatmanesh A, Banaei M, Haghighi KS, Najafi A. Bedroom design orientation and sleep electroencephalography signals. Acta Med Int 2019;6:33-7 http://www.actamedicainternational.com/text.asp?2019/6/1/33/259896

Chapter 4: Nutrients and Foods that promotes better sleep

Melatonin rich foods

1. St-Onge MP, Mikic A, Pietrolungo CE. Effects of Diet on Sleep Quality. *Adv Nutr*. 2016;7(5):938–949. Published 2016 Sep 15. doi:10.3945/an.116.012336

2. Kurdi MS, Muthukalai SP. The Efficacy of Oral Melatonin in Improving Sleep in Cancer Patients with Insomnia: A Randomized Double-Blind Placebo-Controlled Study. *Indian J Palliat Care*. 2016;22(3):295–300. doi:10.4103/0973-1075.185039

3. Wade AG, Ford I, Crawford G, et al. Efficacy of prolonged release melatonin in insomnia patients aged 55-80 years: quality of sleep and next-day alertness outcomes. *Curr Med Res Opin.* 2007;23(10):2597–2605. doi:10.1185/030079907X233098

4. Losso JN, Finley JW, Karki N, et al. Pilot Study of the Tart Cherry Juice for the Treatment of Insomnia and Investigation of Mechanisms. *Am J Ther.* 2018;25(2):e194–e201. doi:10.1097/MJT.0000000000000584

5. Liu, A.Z., Tipton, R., Pan, W., Finley, J.W., Prudente, A., Karki, N., Losso, J.N., & Greenway, F.L. (2014). Experimental Biology, Tart cherry juice increases sleep time in older adults with insomnia (830.9).

6. Howatson G, Bell PG, Tallent J, Middleton B, McHugh MP, Ellis J. Effect of tart cherry juice (Prunus cerasus) on melatonin levels and enhanced sleep quality. *Eur J Nutr.* 2012;51(8):909–916. doi:10.1007/s00394-011-0263-7

7. Pigeon WR, Carr M, Gorman C, Perlis ML. Effects of a tart cherry juice beverage on the sleep of older adults with insomnia: a pilot study. *J Med Food.* 2010;13(3):579–583. doi:10.1089/jmf.2009.0096

8. Lin HH, Tsai PS, Fang SC, Liu JF. Effect of kiwifruit consumption on sleep quality in adults with sleep problems. *Asia Pac J Clin Nutr.* 2011;20(2):169–174.

9. Which foods can help you sleep? Medically reviewed by Katherine Marengo LDN, R.D. Written by Jennifer Huizen, Medical News Today, January 25, 2019

https://www.medicalnewstoday.com/articles/324295

10.Meng X, Li Y, Li S, et al. Dietary Sources and Bioactivities of Melatonin. *Nutrients.* 2017;9(4):367. Published 2017 Apr 7. doi:10.3390/nu9040367

Tryptophan

1. Singh K (2016) Nutrient and Stress Management. J Nutr Food Sci 6: 528. doi:10.4172/2155-9600.1000528

2. Meng X, Li Y, Li S, et al. Dietary Sources and Bioactivities of Melatonin. *Nutrients.* 2017;9(4):367. Published 2017 Apr 7. doi:10.3390/nu9040367

3. https://www.webmd.com/sleep-disorders/ss/slideshow-sleep-foods

4.Coppen A, Eccleston EG, Peet M. Total and free tryptophan concentration in the plasma of depressive patients. *Lancet.* 1973;2(7820):60–63. doi:10.1016/s0140-6736(73)93259-5

5.http://www.vivo.colostate.edu/hbooks/pathphys/endocrine/otherendo/pineal. html

6. Fukushige H, Fukuda Y, Tanaka M, et al. Effects of tryptophan-rich breakfast and light exposure during the daytime on melatonin secretion at night. *J Physiol Anthropol.* 2014;33(1):33. Published 2014 Nov 19. doi:10.1186/1880-6805-33-33

7.Bravo R, Matito S, Cubero J, et al. Tryptophan-enriched cereal intake improves nocturnal sleep, melatonin, serotonin, and total antioxidant capacity levels and mood in elderly humans. *Age (Dordr).* 2013;35(4):1277–1285. doi:10.1007/s11357-012-9419-5

8.Lemoine P, Nir T, Laudon M, Zisapel N. Prolonged-release melatonin improves sleep quality and morning alertness in insomnia patients aged 55 years and older and has no withdrawal effects. *J Sleep Res.* 2007;16(4):372–380. doi:10.1111/j.1365-2869.2007.00613.x

9.https://nutritiondata.self.com/foods-000079000000000000000.html

10. Fernstrom JD. Effects and side effects associated with the non-nutritional use of tryptophan by humans. *J Nutr.* 2012;142(12):2236S–2244S. doi:10.3945/jn.111.157065

11. https://www.sleepfoundation.org/articles/food-and-sleep

12. Gannon MC, Nuttall FQ, Neil BJ, Westphal SA. The insulin and glucoseresponses to meals of glucose plus various proteins in type II diabetic subjects. *Metabolism.* 1988;37(11):1081–1088. doi:10.1016/0026-0495(88)90072-8

13. Gannon MC, Nuttall FQ, Lane JT, Burmeister LA. Metabolic response to cottage cheese or egg white protein, with or without glucose, in type II diabetic subjects. *Metabolism.* 1992;41(10):1137–1145. doi:10.1016/0026-0495(92)90300-y

Magnesium

1.Peuhkuri K, Sihvola N, Korpela R, Dietary factors and fluctuating levels of melatonin, Food Nutr Res.2012;56. doi:10.3402/fnr.v56i0.17252.

2.Meng X, Li Y, Li S, Zhou Y, Gan RY, Xu DP, Li HB., Dietary Sources and Bioactivities of Melatonin, Nutrients. 2017 Apr 7;9(4). pii: E367. doi:10.3390/nu9040367

3.Behnood Abbasi, Masud Kimiagar, Khosro Sadeghniiat, Minoo M. Shirazi, Mehdi Hedayati, and Bahram Rashidkhani,The effect of magnesium supplementation on primary insomnia in elderly: A double-blind placebo-controlled clinical trial, J Res Med Sci. 2012 Dec; 17(12): 1161–1169.

4.Abbasi B, Kimiagar M, Sadeghniiat K, Shirazi MM, Hedayati M, Rashidkhani B., The effect of magnesium supplementation on primary insomnia in elderly: A double-blind placebo-controlled clinical trial, J Res Med Sci. 2012 Dec;17(12):1161-9.

5.Behnood Abbasi, Masud Kimiagar, Khosro Sadeghniiat, Minoo M. Shirazi, Mehdi Hedayati, and Bahram Rashidkhani,The effect of magnesium supplementation on primary insomnia in elderly: A double-blind placebo-controlled clinical trial, J Res Med Sci. 2012 Dec; 17(12): 1161–1169.

6.Rondanelli M, Opizzi A, Monteferrario F, Antoniello N, Manni R, Klersy C.,The effect of melatonin, magnesium, and zinc on primary insomnia in long-term care facility residents in Italy: a double-blind, placebo-controlled clinical trial, J Am Geriatr Soc. 2011 Jan;59(1):82-90. doi: 10.1111/j.1532-5415.2010.03232.x.

7. Insomnia: Studies Suggest Calcium And Magnesium Effective, Medical News Today https://www.medicalnewstoday.com/releases/163169#1

8.https://ods.od.nih.gov/factsheets/Magnesium-HealthProfessional/

B Vitamins

1.Hashimoto S, Kohsaka M, Morita N, Fukuda N, Honma S, Honma K. Vitamin B12 enhances the phase-response of circadian melatonin rhythm to a single bright light exposure in humans. *Neurosci Lett.* 1996;220(2):129–132. doi:10.1016/s0304-3940(96)13247-x.

2.Mayer G, Kröger M, Meier-Ewert K. Effects of vitamin B12 on performance and circadian rhythm in normal subjects. *Neuropsychopharmacology*. 1996;15(5):456–464. doi:10.1016/S0893-133X(96)00055-3

3. St-Onge MP, Mikic A, Pietrolungo CE. Effects of Diet on Sleep Quality. *Adv Nutr*. 2016;7(5):938–949. Published 2016 Sep 15. doi:10.3945/an.116.012336

4. Nutrition's dynamic duos, *Harvard Health Letter* July, 2009

https://www.health.harvard.edu/newsletter_article/Nutritions-dynamic-duos

Calcium and Vitamin D

1.Pablos MI, Agapito MT, Gutierrez-Baraja R, Reiter RJ, Recio JM. Effect of calcium on melatonin secretion in chick pineal gland I. *Neurosci Lett*. 1996;217(2-3):161–164.

2. Insomnia: Studies Suggest Calcium And Magnesium Effective, Medical News Today https://www.medicalnewstoday.com/releases/163169#1

3.St-Onge MP, Mikic A, Pietrolungo CE. Effects of Diet on Sleep Quality. *Adv Nutr*. 2016;7(5):938–949. Published 2016 Sep 15. doi:10.3945/an.116.012336

4.Gao Q, Kou T, Zhuang B, Ren Y, Dong X, Wang Q. The Association between Vitamin D Deficiency and Sleep Disorders: A Systematic Review and Meta-Analysis. *Nutrients*. 2018;10(10):1395. Published 2018 Oct 1. doi:10.3390/nu10101395

5.https://ods.od.nih.gov/factsheets/VitaminD-HealthProfessional/

6. https://ods.od.nih.gov/factsheets/VitaminD-Consumer/

Chamomile Tea

1.Srivastava JK, Shankar E, Gupta S. Chamomile: A herbal medicine of the past with bright future. *Mol Med Rep*. 2010;3(6):895–901. doi:10.3892/mmr.2010.377

2.Zick SM, Wright BD, Sen A, Arnedt JT. Preliminary examination of the efficacy and safety of a standardized chamomile extract for chronic primary insomnia: a randomized placebo-controlled pilot study. *BMC Complement Altern Med.* 2011;11:78. Published 2011 Sep 22. doi:10.1186/1472-6882-11-78

3.GOULD, L., REDDY, C.V.R. and GOMPRECHT, R.F. (1973), Cardiac Effects of Chamomile Tea. The Journal of Clinical Pharmacology and New Drugs, 13: 475-479. doi:10.1002/j.1552-4604.1973.tb00202.x

4.Srivastava JK, Shankar E, Gupta S. Chamomile: A herbal medicine of the past with bright future. *Mol Med Rep.* 2010;3(6):895–901. doi:10.3892/mmr.2010.377

5.Chang SM, Chen CH. Effects of an intervention with drinking chamomile tea on sleep quality and depression in sleep disturbed postnatal women: a randomized controlled trial. *J Adv Nurs.* 2016;72(2):306–315. doi:10.1111/jan.12836

6.Leach MJ, Page AT. Herbal medicine for insomnia: A systematic review and meta-analysis. *Sleep Med Rev.* 2015;24:1–12. doi:10.1016/j.smrv.2014.12.003

7.Adib-Hajbaghery M, Mousavi SN. The effects of chamomile extract on sleep quality among elderly people: A clinical trial. *Complement Ther Med.* 2017;35:109–114. doi:10.1016/j.ctim.2017.09.010

8.https://www.webmd.com/diet/supplement-guide-chamomile#1

Fatty Fish

1.Patrick RP, Ames BN. Vitamin D and the omega-3 fatty acids control serotonin synthesis and action, part 2: relevance for ADHD, bipolar disorder, schizophrenia, and impulsive behavior. *FASEB J.* 2015;29(6):2207–2222. doi:10.1096/fj.14-268342

2.St-Onge MP, Mikic A, Pietrolungo CE. Effects of Diet on Sleep Quality. *Adv Nutr.* 2016;7(5):938–949. Published 2016 Sep 15. doi:10.3945/an.116.012336

3.Grosso G, Galvano F, Marventano S, et al. Omega-3 fatty acids and depression: scientific evidence and biological mechanisms. *Oxid Med Cell Longev.* 2014;2014:313570. doi:10.1155/2014/313570

4.Hansen AL, Dahl L, Olson G, et al. Fish consumption, sleep, daily functioning, and heart rate variability. *J Clin Sleep Med.* 2014;10(5):567–575. doi:10.5664/jcsm.3714

5.Hansen AL, Olson G, Dahl L, et al. Reduced anxiety in forensic inpatients after a long-term intervention with Atlantic salmon. *Nutrients.* 2014;6(12):5405–5418. Published 2014 Nov 26. doi:10.3390/nu6125405

Barley grass powder

1.Zeng Y, Pu X, Yang J, et al. Preventive and Therapeutic Role of Functional Ingredients of Barley Grass for Chronic Diseases in Human Beings. *Oxid Med Cell Longev.* 2018;2018:3232080. Published 2018 Apr 4. doi:10.1155/2018/3232080

2. https://www.drugs.com/npc/barley-grass.html

Lettuce

1.Kim HD, Hong KB, Noh DO, Suh HJ. Sleep-inducing effect of lettuce (*Lactuca sativa*) varieties on pentobarbital-induced sleep. *Food Sci Biotechnol.* 2017;26(3):807–814. Published 2017 May 29. doi:10.1007/s10068-017-0107-1

2. Hong KB, Han SH, Park Y, Suh HJ, Choi HS. Romaine Lettuce/Skullcap Mixture Improves Sleep Behavior in Vertebrate Models. *Biol Pharm Bull.* 2018;41(8):1269–1276. doi:10.1248/bpb.b18-00267

3.Pour ZS, Hosseinkhani A, Asadi N, et al. Double-blind randomized placebo-controlled trial on efficacy and safety of Lactuca sativa L. seeds on pregnancy-related insomnia. *J Ethnopharmacol.* 2018;227:176–180. doi:10.1016/j.jep.2018.08.001

4.Yakoot M, Helmy S, Fawal K. Pilot study of the efficacy and safety of lettuce seed oil in patients with sleep disorders. *Int J Gen Med.* 2011;4:451–456. doi:10.2147/IJGM.S21529

Chapter 5: Macronutrients on sleep: Carbohydrates, Protein and Fats

1.Lindseth G, Murray A. Dietary Macronutrients and Sleep. *West J Nurs Res*. 2016;38(8):938–958. doi:10.1177/0193945916643712

2. Shi Z, McEvoy M, Luu J, Attia J. Dietary fat and sleep duration in Chinese men and women. *Int J Obes (Lond)*. 2008;32(12):1835–1840. doi:10.1038/ijo.2008.191

3. American Academy of Sleep Medicine. "What you eat can influence how you sleep: Daily intake of fiber, saturated fat and sugar may impact sleep quality." ScienceDaily. ScienceDaily, 14 January 2016. <www.sciencedaily.com/releases/2016/01/160114213443.htm>.

4 Hallböök T, Lundgren J, Rosén I. Ketogenic diet improves sleep quality in children with therapy-resistant epilepsy. *Epilepsia*. 2007;48(1):59–65. doi:10.1111/j.1528-1167.2006.00834.x

5.Afaghi A, O'Connor H, Chow CM. Acute effects of the very low carbohydrate diet on sleep indices. *Nutr Neurosci*. 2008;11(4):146–154. doi:10.1179/147683008X301540

6. Schmidt M, Pfetzer N, Schwab M, Strauss I, Kämmerer U. Effects of a ketogenic diet on the quality of life in 16 patients with advanced cancer: A pilot trial. *Nutr Metab (Lond)*. 2011;8(1):54. Published 2011 Jul 27. doi:10.1186/1743-7075-8-54

7.Lindseth G, Murray A. Dietary Macronutrients and Sleep. *West J Nurs Res*. 2016;38(8):938–958. doi:10.1177/0193945916643712

8. Unger, A.L.; Torres-Gonzalez, M.; Kraft, J. Dairy Fat Consumption and the Risk of Metabolic Syndrome: An Examination of the Saturated Fatty Acids in Dairy. *Nutrients* 2019, *11*, 2200.

9. Drouin-Chartier JP, Côté JA, Labonté MÈ, et al. Comprehensive Review of the Impact of Dairy Foods and Dairy Fat on Cardiometabolic Risk. *Adv Nutr*. 2016;7(6):1041-1051. Published 2016 Nov 15. doi:10.3945/an.115.011619

10.Sutanto, C.N.; Wang, M.X.; Tan, D.; Kim, J.E. Association of Sleep Quality and Macronutrient Distribution: A Systematic Review and Meta-Regression. *Nutrients* 2020, *12*, 126

11. American Academy of Sleep Medicine. "What you eat can influence how you sleep: Daily intake of fiber, saturated fat and sugar may impact sleep quality." ScienceDaily. ScienceDaily, 14 January 2016. <www.sciencedaily.com/releases/2016/01/160114213443.htm>.

12. St-Onge MP, Mikic A, Pietrolungo CE. Effects of Diet on Sleep Quality. *Adv Nutr.* 2016;7(5):938–949. Published 2016 Sep 15. doi:10.3945/an.116.012336

13. Zhou J, Kim JE, Armstrong CL, Chen N, Campbell WW. Higher-protein diets improve indexes of sleep in energy-restricted overweight and obese adults: results from 2 randomized controlled trials. *Am J Clin Nutr.* 2016;103(3):766–774. doi:10.3945/ajcn.115.124669

14.Donald K Layman, Tracy G Anthony, Blake B Rasmussen, Sean H Adams, Christopher J Lynch, Grant D Brinkworth, and Teresa A Davis, Defining meal requirements for protein to optimize metabolic roles of amino acids⋅ Am J Clin Nutr. 2015 Jun; 101(6): 1330S–1338S,

15. How much protein do you need every day?,Daniel Pendick, Harvard Health Publishing, JUNE 25, 2019 https://www.health.harvard.edu/blog/how-much-protein-do-you-need-every-day-201506188096

16. "How much protein do you need per day?," Examine.com, published on 16 January 2013, last updated on 5 July 2020, https://examine.com/nutrition/how-much-protein-do-you-need/

17.Gangwisch JE, Hale L, St-Onge MP, et al. High glycemic index and glycemic load diets as risk factors for insomnia: analyses from the Women's Health Initiative. *Am J Clin Nutr.* 2020;111(2):429–439. doi:10.1093/ajcn/nqz275

18.Spring B. Recent research on the behavioral effects of tryptophan and carbohydrate. *Nutr Health.* 1984;3(1-2):55–67. doi:10.1177/026010608400300204

19.Wurtman RJ, Wurtman JJ. Carbohydrate craving, obesity and brain serotonin. *Appetite.* 1986;7 Suppl:99–103. doi:10.1016/s0195-6663(86)80055-1

20.Lindseth G, Murray A. Dietary Macronutrients and Sleep. *West J Nurs Res.* 2016;38(8):938–958. doi:10.1177/0193945916643712

Chapter 6: Night time foods that can hurt your sleep

1.Shaun F.Morrison, Handbook of Clinical Neurology, 2018 https://www.sciencedirect.com/topics/psychology/adenosine

2. Sheth S, Brito R, Mukherjea D, Rybak LP, Ramkumar V. Adenosine receptors: expression, function and regulation. *Int J Mol Sci*. 2014;15(2):2024–2052. Published 2014 Jan 28. doi:10.3390/ijms15022024

3.Cunha RA. Adenosine as a neuromodulator and as a homeostatic regulator in the nervous system: different roles, different sources and different receptors. *Neurochem Int*. 2001;38(2):107–125. doi:10.1016/s0197-0186(00)00034-6

4.Bjorness TE, Greene RW. Adenosine and sleep. *Curr Neuropharmacol*. 2009;7(3):238–245. doi:10.2174/157015909789152182

5. Huang ZL, Urade Y, Hayaishi O. The role of adenosine in the regulation of sleep. *Curr Top Med Chem*. 2011;11(8):1047–1057. doi:10.2174/156802611795347654

6. Porkka-Heiskanen T, Alanko L, Kalinchuk A, Stenberg D. Adenosine and sleep. *Sleep Med Rev*. 2002;6(4):321–332. doi:10.1053/smrv.2001.0201

7. Ribeiro JA, Sebastião AM. Caffeine and adenosine. *J Alzheimers Dis*. 2010;20 Suppl 1:S3–S15. doi:10.3233/JAD-2010-1379

8. Snel J, Lorist MM. Effects of caffeine on sleep and cognition. *Prog Brain Res*. 2011;190:105–117. doi:10.1016/B978-0-444-53817-8.00006-2

9. Drake C, Roehrs T, Shambroom J, Roth T. Caffeine effects on sleep taken 0, 3, or 6 hours before going to bed. *J Clin Sleep Med*. 2013;9(11):1195–1200. Published 2013 Nov 15. doi:10.5664/jcsm.3170

10.Roehrs T, Roth T. Caffeine: sleep and daytime sleepiness. *Sleep Med Rev*. 2008;12(2):153–162. doi:10.1016/j.smrv.2007.07.004

11. 10 Healthy Herbal Teas You Should Try, by Taylor Jones, RD, Healthline, October 20, 2017,https://www.healthline.com/nutrition/10-herbal-teas

12. Cohen MM. Tulsi - Ocimum sanctum: A herb for all reasons. *J Ayurveda Integr Med*. 2014;5(4):251–259. doi:10.4103/0975-9476.146554

13. Fadaki F, Modaresi M, Sajjadian I. The Effects of Ginger Extract and Diazepam on Anxiety Reduction in Animal Model. Indian J of Pharmaceutical Education and Research. 2017;51(3)Suppl:S159-62.

14. Nutritional strategies to ease anxiety, Uma Naidoo, MD, Harvard Health Publishing, August 29, 2019 https://www.health.harvard.edu/blog/nutritional-strategies-to-ease-anxiety-201604139441

15. Nievergelt A, Huonker P, Schoop R, Altmann KH, Gertsch J. Identification of serotonin 5-HT1A receptor partial agonists in ginger. *Bioorg Med Chem.* 2010;18(9):3345–3351. doi:10.1016/j.bmc.2010.02.062

16. Health benefits of peppermint tea,Medically reviewed by Katherine Marengo LDN, R.D. — Written by Jenna Fletcher, Medical News Today, May 22, 2019, https://www.medicalnewstoday.com/articles/325242

17. Chandini Ravikumar /J. Pharm. Sci. & Res. Vol. 6(5), 2014, 236-238

18.   https://www.sleepfoundation.org/articles/food-and-drink-promote-good-nights-sleep

19.https://www.myfooddata.com/articles/high-caffeine-foods-and-drinks.php

20. Surprising Foods That Contain Caffeine, National Sleep Foundation, https://www.sleep.org/articles/foods-with-caffeine/

21.Tyramine, MIGRAINE AND DIET, *M.R. Costa, M.B.A. Glória, in* Encyclopedia of Food Sciences and Nutrition (Second Edition)*, 2003,* https://doi.org/10.1016/B0-12-227055-X/00783-5

https://www.sciencedirect.com/science/article/pii/B012227055X007835

22. Sathyanarayana Rao TS, Yeragani VK. Hypertensive crisis and cheese. *Indian J Psychiatry.* 2009;51(1):65–66. doi:10.4103/0019-5545.44910

23. Tyramine and Migraines, Reviewed by Jennifer Robinson, MD, WebMD on August 18, 2018https://www.webmd.com/migraines-headaches/tyramine-and-migraines#1

24. Ghose K, Coppen A, Carrol D. Intravenous tyramine response in migraine before and during treatment with indoramin. Br Med J 1977; 1 :1191, doi: https://doi.org/10.1136/bmj.1.6070.1191

25. MAOIs and diet: Is it necessary to restrict tyramine? Daniel K. Hall-Flavin, M.D.   ,   Mayo   Clinic   https://www.mayoclinic.org/diseases-conditions/depression/expert-answers/maois/faq-20058035

26. Tyramine and Migraines, Reviewed by Jennifer Robinson, MD, WebMD on August 18, 2018https://www.webmd.com/migraines-headaches/tyramine-and-migraines#1

27.https://www.sleepfoundation.org/articles/food-and-drink-promote-good-nights-sleep

28. Guide to Natural Diuretics, Medically reviewed by Carissa Stephens, RN, CCRN, CPN — Written by Colleen M. Story — Healthline, May 11, 2019, https://www.healthline.com/health/natural-diuretics#prescription-diuretics

29. https://www.webmd.com/vitamins/ai/ingredientmono-545/lemon

30. 9 Fruits and Vegetables That Are Natural Diuretics, BY STEPHANIE FEUER, Good Housekeeping, Sep 4, 2018 https://www.goodhousekeeping.com/health/diet-nutrition/a20707480/natural-diuretics/

31. Lopes TVC, Borba ME, Lopes RVC, Fisberg RM, Paim SL, Teodoro VV, Zimberg IZ, Crispim CA. Eating late negatively affects sleep pattern and apnea severity in individuals with sleep apnea. *J Clin Sleep Med.* 2019;15(3):383–392. https://doi.org/10.5664/jcsm.7658

32. Crispim CA, Zimberg IZ, dos Reis BG, Diniz RM, Tufik S, de Mello MT. Relationship between food intake and sleep pattern in healthy individuals. *J Clin Sleep Med.* 2011;7(6):659–664. doi:10.5664/jcsm.1476

33. https://www.nhlbi.nih.gov/files/docs/public/sleep/healthysleepfs.pdf

34. American Academy of Sleep Medicine. "What you eat can influence how you sleep: Daily intake of fiber, saturated fat and sugar may impact sleep quality." ScienceDaily. ScienceDaily, 14 January 2016. <www.sciencedaily.com/releases/2016/01/160114213443.htm>.

35.Plataforma SINC. "Fried food risks: Toxic aldehydes detected in reheated oil." ScienceDaily. ScienceDaily, 22 February 2012. <www.sciencedaily.com/releases/2012/02/120222093508.htm>.

36.Sullivan EV, Harris RA, Pfefferbaum A. Alcohol's effects on brain and behavior. *Alcohol Res Health.* 2010;33(1-2):127–143

37. Blum K, Thanos PK, Gold MS. Dopamine and glucose, obesity, and reward deficiency syndrome. *Front Psychol.* 2014;5:919. Published 2014 Sep 17. doi:10.3389/fpsyg.2014.00919

38.Zahr NM, Pfefferbaum A. Alcohol's Effects on the Brain: Neuroimaging Results in Humans and Animal Models. *Alcohol Res*. 2017;38(2):183–206.

39. Alcohol and a Good Night's Sleep Don't Mix, Denise Mann, WebMD https://www.webmd.com/sleep-disorders/news/20130118/alcohol-sleep#1

40.Rupp TL, Acebo C, Carskadon MA. Evening alcohol suppresses salivary melatonin in young adults. *Chronobiol Int*. 2007;24(3):463–470. doi:10.1080/07420520701420675

41. Leary EB, Watson KT, Ancoli-Israel S, et al. Association of Rapid Eye Movement Sleep With Mortality in Middle-aged and Older Adults. *JAMA Neurol*. Published online July 06, 2020. doi:10.1001/jamaneurol.2020.2108

Chapter 7: Gut health

1.Thursby E, Juge N. Introduction to the human gut microbiota. *Biochem J*. 2017;474(11):1823-1836. Published 2017 May 16. doi:10.1042/BCJ20160510

2.Wallace CJK, Milev R. The effects of probiotics on depressive symptoms in humans: a systematic review [published correction appears in Ann Gen Psychiatry. 2017 Mar 7;16:18]. *Ann Gen Psychiatry*. 2017;16:14. Published 2017 Feb 20. doi:10.1186/s12991-017-0138-2

3.Health benefits of taking probiotics, Harvard Health Publishing, April 13, 2020

https://www.health.harvard.edu/vitamins-and-supplements/health-benefits-of-taking-probiotics

4.Dimidi E, Cox SR, Rossi M, Whelan K. Fermented Foods: Definitions and Characteristics, Impact on the Gut Microbiota and Effects on Gastrointestinal Health and Disease. *Nutrients*. 2019;11(8):1806. Published 2019 Aug 5. doi:10.3390/nu11081806

5.Pei R, DiMarco DM, Putt KK, et al. Premeal Low-Fat Yogurt Consumption Reduces Postprandial Inflammation and Markers of Endotoxin Exposure in Healthy Premenopausal Women in a Randomized Controlled Trial [published correction appears in J Nutr. 2018 Oct 1;148(10):1698]. *J Nutr*. 2018;148(6):910-916. doi:10.1093/jn/nxy046

6.Han K, Bose S, Wang JH, et al. Contrasting effects of fresh and fermented kimchi consumption on gut microbiota composition and gene expression related to metabolic syndrome in obese Korean women. *Mol Nutr Food Res*. 2015;59(5):1004-1008. doi:10.1002/mnfr.201400780

7.Kil, J.-H., Jung, K.-O., Lee, H.-S., Hwang, I.-K., Kim, Y.-J., & Park, K.-Y. (2004). Effects of Kimchi on Stomach and Colon Health of Helicobacter pylori-Infected Volunteers. *Preventive Nutrition and Food Science* , 9 (2), 161–166. https://doi.org/10.3746/jfn.2004.9.2.161

8.Rezac S, Kok CR, Heermann M, Hutkins R. Fermented Foods as a Dietary Source of Live Organisms. *Front Microbiol*. 2018;9:1785. Published 2018 Aug 24. doi:10.3389/fmicb.2018.01785

9.Melini F, Melini V, Luziatelli F, Ficca AG, Ruzzi M. Health-Promoting Components in Fermented Foods: An Up-to-Date Systematic Review. *Nutrients*. 2019;11(5):1189. Published 2019 May 27. doi:10.3390/nu11051189

10.Cummings JH, Macfarlane GT. Gastrointestinal effects of prebiotics. *Br J Nutr*. 2002;87 Suppl 2:S145-S151. doi:10.1079/BJNBJN/2002530

11. Macfarlane GT, Steed H, Macfarlane S. Bacterial metabolism and health-related effects of galacto-oligosaccharides and other prebiotics. *J Appl Microbiol*. 2008;104(2):305-344. doi:10.1111/j.1365-2672.2007.03520.x

12. Slavin J. Fiber and prebiotics: mechanisms and health benefits. *Nutrients*. 2013;5(4):1417-1435. Published 2013 Apr 22. doi:10.3390/nu5041417

13. Kakodkar S, Mutlu EA. Diet as a Therapeutic Option for Adult Inflammatory Bowel Disease. *Gastroenterol Clin North Am*. 2017;46(4):745–767. doi:10.1016/j.gtc.2017.08.016

14.Lladó S, López-Mondéjar R, Baldrian P. Forest Soil Bacteria: Diversity, Involvement in Ecosystem Processes, and Response to Global Change. *Microbiol Mol Biol Rev*. 2017;81(2):e00063-16. Published 2017 Apr 12. doi:10.1128/MMBR.00063-16

15.Craig JM, Logan AC, Prescott SL. Natural environments, nature relatedness and the ecological theater: connecting satellites and sequencing to shinrin-yoku. *J Physiol Anthropol*. 2016;35:1. Published 2016 Jan 13. doi:10.1186/s40101-016-0083-9

Chapter 8: Effect of light, color, temperature and noise in Bedroom

1. Light-Emitting E-Readers Before Bedtime Can Adversely Impact Sleep, Brigham and Women's Hospital, December 22, 2014 https://www.brighamandwomens.org/about-bwh/newsroom/press-releases-detail?id=1962

2. Blue light has a dark side, Harvard Health Letter, July 7, 2020https://www.health.harvard.edu/staying-healthy/blue-light-has-a-dark-side

3. Yoneyama S, Sakurai M, Nakamura K, et al. Associations between rice, noodle, and bread intake and sleep quality in Japanese men and women. *PLoS One.* 2014;9(8):e105198. Published 2014 Aug 15. doi:10.1371/journal.pone.0105198

4. https://www.sleep.org/articles/temperature-for-sleep/

Chapter 9: Activities that can hurt your sleep

Stop nap after 3 pm

1. Your Guide to Healthy Sleep, NHLBI Health Information Center, September, 2011 https://www.nhlbi.nih.gov/files/docs/public/sleep/healthysleepfs.pdf

Bedtime use of cell phone/tablets

1.Blue light has a dark side, Harvard Health Publishing, July 7, 2020 https://www.health.harvard.edu/staying-healthy/blue-light-has-a-dark-side

2.Will blue light from electronic devices increase my risk of macular degeneration and blindness? David Ramsey, MD, PhD, MPH, Harvard Health Publishing, MAY 01, 2019, https://www.health.harvard.edu/blog/will-blue-light-from-electronic-devices-increase-my-risk-of-macular-degeneration-and-blindness-2019040816365

3.Three ways gadgets are keeping you awake, National Sleep Foundation, https://www.sleep.org/articles/ways-technology-affects-sleep/

4.Lee SI, Matsumori K, Nishimura K, et al. Melatonin suppression and sleepiness in children exposed to blue-enriched white LED lighting at night. *Physiol Rep.* 2018;6(24):e13942. doi:10.14814/phy2.13942 https://www.ncbi.nlm.nih.gov/pmc/articles/PMC6295443/

5.How Electronics Affect Sleep, National Sleep Foundation, July 28, 2020 https://www.sleepfoundation.org/bedroom-environment/see/how-electronics-affect-sleep

6.Put the Phone Away! 3 Reasons Why Looking at It Before Bed Is a Bad Habit, April 22, 2019, Cleveland Clinic https://health.clevelandclinic.org/put-the-phone-away-3-reasons-why-looking-at-it-before-bed-is-a-bad-habit/

7.6 Ways That Night-time Phone Use Destroys Your Sleep, Susan Biali Haas M.D., Psychology Today, Apr 17, 2018, https://www.psychologytoday.com/intl/blog/prescriptions-life/201804/6-ways-night-time-phone-use-destroys-your-sleep

8. Rasch B, Born J. About sleep's role in memory. *Physiol Rev.* 2013;93(2):681-766. doi:10.1152/physrev.00032.2012 https://www.ncbi.nlm.nih.gov/pmc/articles/PMC3768102/

9.Why Electronics May Stimulate You Before Bed, The National Sleep Foundation, July 28, 2020 https://www.sleepfoundation.org/articles/why-electronics-may-stimulate-you-bed

Should you do exercise before bedtime?

1. Can Exercising at Night Hurt Your Sleep? By Tom DiChiara, WebMD, https://www.webmd.com/sleep-disorders/features/can-exercising-at-night-hurt-your-sleep#1

2.Stutz J, Eiholzer R, Spengler CM. Effects of Evening Exercise on Sleep in Healthy Participants: A Systematic Review and Meta-Analysis. *Sports Med.* 2019;49(2):269–287. doi:10.1007/s40279-018-1015-0

3. Does exercising at night affect sleep? by Howard LeWine, M.D. Editor in Chief, Harvard Men's Health Watch, April, 2019 https://www.health.harvard.edu/staying-healthy/does-exercising-at-night-affect-sleep

4.Wang F, Eun-Kyoung Lee O, Feng F, et al. The effect of meditative movement on sleep quality: A systematic review. *Sleep Med Rev.* 2016;30:43–52. doi:10.1016/j.smrv.2015.12.001

5.https://www.sleep.org/articles/nighttime-exercise-routines/

How good watching TV before bed for sleep?

1. Light-Emitting E-Readers Before Bedtime Can Adversely Impact Sleep, Brigham and Women's Hospital, December 22, 2014 https://www.brighamandwomens.org/about-bwh/newsroom/press-releases-detail?id=1962

2. Blue light has a dark side, What is blue light? The effect blue light has on your sleep and more, Harvard Health Publishing, August 13, 2018, https://www.health.harvard.edu/staying-healthy/blue-light-has-a-dark-side

3.Wood B, Rea MS, Plitnick B, Figueiro MG. Light level and duration of exposure determine the impact of self-luminous tablets on melatonin suppression. *Appl Ergon.* 2013;44(2):237–240. doi:10.1016/j.apergo.2012.07.008

4. https://www.sleep.org/articles/is-it-bad-to-watch-tv-right-before-bed/

5. Why Watching TV Re-Runs Helps Ease Stress, By Elizabeth Scott, MS, Verywell Mind, August 04, 2019,https://www.verywellmind.com/the-surprising-benefits-of-re-runs-3144586

6. Mesquita, Gema, & Reimão, Rubens. (2010). Quality of sleep among university students: effects of nighttime computer and television use. *Arquivos de Neuro-Psiquiatria, 68*(5), 720-725. https://doi.org/10.1590/S0004-282X2010000500009

7.https://www.sleep.org/articles/is-it-bad-to-watch-tv-right-before-bed/

Eliminate electromagnetic fields (EMFs) from your bedroom

1. Pall ML. Microwave frequency electromagnetic fields (EMFs) produce widespread neuropsychiatric effects including depression. *J Chem Neuroanat.* 2016;75(Pt B):43–51. doi:10.1016/j.jchemneu.2015.08.001

2.Barsam T, Monazzam MR, Haghdoost AA, Ghotbi MR, Dehghan SF. Effect of extremely low frequency electromagnetic field exposure on sleep quality in high voltage substations. *Iranian J Environ Health Sci Eng.* 2012;9(1):15. Published 2012 Nov 30. doi:10.1186/1735-2746-9-15

Chapter 10: Strategies for going to bed

1.Levenson JC, Shensa A, Sidani JE, Colditz JB, Primack BA. The association between social media use and sleep disturbance among young adults. *Prev Med.* 2016;85:36-41. doi:10.1016/j.ypmed.2016.01.001

2.Levenson JC, Shensa A, Sidani JE, Colditz JB, Primack BA. Social Media Use Before Bed and Sleep Disturbance Among Young Adults in the United States: A Nationally Representative Study. *Sleep.* 2017;40(9):10.1093/sleep/zsx113. doi:10.1093/sleep/zsx113

3.University of Texas at Austin. "Take a bath 90 minutes before bedtime to get better sleep." ScienceDaily. ScienceDaily, 19 July 2019. <www.sciencedaily.com/releases/2019/07/190719173554.htm>

4. Shahab Haghayegh, Sepideh Khoshnevis, Michael H. Smolensky, Kenneth R. Diller, Richard J. Castriotta. Before-bedtime passive body heating by warm shower or bath to improve sleep: A systematic review and meta-analysis. *Sleep Medicine Reviews,* 2019; 46: 124 DOI: 10.1016/j.smrv.2019.04.008

5. When's the best time to take a warm bath for better sleep? by Ana Sandoiu, fact checked by Jasmin Collier, Medical News Today, July 22, 2019, https://www.medicalnewstoday.com/articles/325818#Analyzing-bathing-time-and-sleep-quality

6.http://nationalreadingcampaign.ca/wp-content/uploads/2013/09/ReadingFacts1.pdf

7.https://www.takingcharge.csh.umn.edu/reading-stress-relief

8.Hughes TF, Chang CC, Vander Bilt J, Ganguli M. Engagement in reading and hobbies and risk of incident dementia: the MoVIES project. *Am J Alzheimers Dis Other Demen.* 2010;25(5):432-438. doi:10.1177/1533317510368399

9.https://www.comvita.com/blog-article/how-reading-can-reduce-stress/400323

10.https://www.sleepfoundation.org/articles/why-electronics-may-stimulate-you-bed

11.https://www.sleep.org/articles/wearing-socks-to-bed/

Chapter 11: Stress handling

1. Han KS, Kim L, Shim I. Stress and sleep disorder. *Exp Neurobiol.* 2012;21(4):141-150. doi:10.5607/en.2012.21.4.141

2.Jackson, Erica M. Ph.D., FACSM, STRESS RELIEF: The Role of Exercise in Stress Management, ACSM's Health & Fitness Journal: May/June 2013 - Volume 17 - Issue 3 - p 14-19, doi: 10.1249/FIT.0b013e31828cb1c9

3.Stress Management, by Lawrence Robinson, Melinda Smith, M.A., and Robert Segal, M.A., October 2019, Helpguide https://www.helpguide.org/articles/stress/stress-management.htm

Chapter 12: Why Exercise? Way to include exercise in daily routine

1.Dopamine and serotonin: Brain chemicals explained, Medically reviewed by Heidi Moawad, M.D. — Written by Jamie Eske, Medical News Today, August 19, 2019, https://www.medicalnewstoday.com/articles/326090

2.What is Serotonin? Irina Bancos, M.D, The Hormone Health Network December 2018 https://www.hormone.org/your-health-and-hormones/glands-and-hormones-a-to-z/hormones/serotonin

3. Norepinephrine, Eleni Dimaraki, M.D., MS, September 2019, The Hormone Health Network https://www.hormone.org/your-health-and-hormones/glands-and-hormones-a-to-z/hormones/norepinephrine

4.Kuo YM. Exercise benefits brain function: the monoamine connection. *Brain Sci.* 2013;3(1):39-53. Published 2013 Jan 11. doi:10.3390/brainsci3010039

5.Exercise, Depression, and the Brain, Medically reviewed by Timothy J. Legg, PMHNP-BC, GNP-BC, CARN-AP, MCHES — Written by Ryan Collins, Healthline July 25, 2017 https://www.healthline.com/health/depression/exercise#1

6.Babyak M, Blumenthal JA, Herman S, et al. Exercise treatment for major depression: maintenance of therapeutic benefit at 10 months. *Psychosom Med.* 2000;62(5):633-638. doi:10.1097/00006842-200009000-00006

7.Kuo YM. Exercise benefits brain function: the monoamine connection. *Brain Sci.* 2013;3(1):39-53. Published 2013 Jan 11. doi:10.3390/brainsci3010039

8.Hillman CH, Erickson KI, Kramer AF. Be smart, exercise your heart: exercise effects on brain and cognition. *Nat Rev Neurosci.* 2008;9(1):58-65. doi:10.1038/nrn2298

9.Preventing Alzheimer's Disease, *Melinda Smith, M.A., Lawrence Robinson, and Jeanne Segal, Ph.D.* HelpGuide, *February 2020* https://www.helpguide.org/articles/alzheimers-dementia-aging/preventing-alzheimers-disease.htm

10.Dorling J, Broom DR, Burns SF, et al. Acute and Chronic Effects of Exercise on Appetite, Energy Intake, and Appetite-Related Hormones: The Modulating Effect of Adiposity, Sex, and Habitual Physical Activity. *Nutrients.* 2018;10(9):1140. Published 2018 Aug 22. doi:10.3390/nu10091140

11. Can Exercising at Night Hurt Your Sleep? By Tom DiChiara, WebMD https://www.webmd.com/sleep-disorders/features/can-exercising-at-night-hurt-your-sleep#2

12.Buman MP, Phillips BA, Youngstedt SD, Kline CE, Hirshkowitz M. Does nighttime exercise really disturb sleep? Results from the 2013 National Sleep Foundation Sleep in America Poll. *Sleep Med.* 2014;15(7):755–761. doi:10.1016/j.sleep.2014.01.008

13.Stutz J, Eiholzer R, Spengler CM. Effects of Evening Exercise on Sleep in Healthy Participants: A Systematic Review and Meta-Analysis. *Sports Med.* 2019;49(2):269–287. doi:10.1007/s40279-018-1015-0

14. Does exercising at night affect sleep? by Howard LeWine, M.D. Editor in Chief, Harvard Men's Health Watch, April, 2019 https://www.health.harvard.edu/staying-healthy/does-exercising-at-night-affect-sleep

15..Stults-Kolehmainen MA, Sinha R. The effects of stress on physical activity and exercise. *Sports Med.* 2014;44(1):81–121. doi:10.1007/s40279-013-0090-5

16.Van Proeyen K, Szlufcik K, Nielens H, et al. Training in the fasted state improves glucose tolerance during fat-rich diet. *J Physiol.* 2010;588(Pt 21):4289-4302. doi:10.1113/jphysiol.2010.196493

17.How much should the average adult exercise every day? Answer from Edward R. Laskowski, M.D., April 27, 2019, Mayo Clinic https://www.mayoclinic.org/healthy-lifestyle/fitness/expert-answers/exercise/faq-20057916

18.Jackson, Erica M. Ph.D., FACSM, STRESS RELIEF: The Role of Exercise in Stress Management, ACSM's Health & Fitness Journal: May/June 2013 - Volume 17 - Issue 3 - p 14-19, doi: 10.1249/FIT.0b013e31828cb1c9

19. Strength and Resistance Training Exercise, American Heart Association, Apr 19, 2018 https://www.heart.org/en/healthy-living/fitness/fitness-basics/strength-and-resistance-training-exercise#.VtS9lhh1bYI

20.Seguin R, Nelson ME. The benefits of strength training for older adults. *Am J Prev Med.* 2003;25(3 Suppl 2):141–149. doi:10.1016/s0749-3797(03)00177-6

21..Fragala, Maren S., Cadore, Eduardo L.,Dorgo, Sandol, Izquierdo, Mikel, Kraemer, William J., Peterson, Mark D., Ryan, Eric D., Resistance Training for Older Adults, Position Statement From the National Strength and Conditioning Association, The Journal of Strength & Conditioning Research: August 2019 - Volume 33 - Issue 8 - p 2019-2052 doi: 10.1519/JSC.0000000000003230

22.https://www.cdc.gov/physicalactivity/downloads/growing_stronger.pdf

23. Nishigawa K, Suzuki Y, Matsuka Y. Masticatory performance alters stress relief effect of gum chewing. *J Prosthodont Res.* 2015;59(4):262-267. doi:10.1016/j.jpor.2015.07.004

24. Smith AP. Chewing gum and stress reduction. *J Clin Transl Res.* 2016;2(2):52-54. Published 2016 Apr 24.

Chapter 13: Strategy for wellbeing in life

1.Berwick DM. The Moral Determinants of Health. *JAMA.* Published online June 12, 2020. doi:10.1001/jama.2020.11129 https://jamanetwork.com/journals/jama/fullarticle/2767353?

2. Nickerson C, Schwarz N, Diener E, Kahneman D. Zeroing in on the dark side of the American Dream: a closer look at the negative consequences of the goal for financial success. Psychol Sci. 2003 Nov;14(6):531-6. doi: 10.1046/j.0956-7976.2003.psci_1461.x. PMID: 14629682. https://pubmed.ncbi.nlm.nih.gov/14629682/

3.Lyubomirsky, S., Sheldon, K. M., & Schkade, D. (2005). Pursuing Happiness: The Architecture of Sustainable Change. Review of General Psychology, 9(2), 111–131. https://doi.org/10.1037/1089-2680.9.2.111

4.Lyubomirsky S, Dickerhoof R, Boehm JK, Sheldon KM. Becoming happier takes both a will and a proper way: an experimental longitudinal intervention to boost wellbeing. *Emotion.* 2011;11(2):391-402. doi:10.1037/a0022575

5.https://www.edbatista.com/2009/02/happiness.html

6.Lucas RE, Clark AE, Georgellis Y, Diener E. Reexamining adaptation and the set point model of happiness: reactions to changes in marital status. J Pers Soc Psychol. 2003 Mar;84(3):527-39. doi: 10.1037//0022-3514.84.3.527. PMID: 12635914. https://pubmed.ncbi.nlm.nih.gov/12635914/

7. https://en.wikipedia.org/wiki/Mike_Tyson

8.https://en.wikipedia.org/wiki/Cus_D%27Amato

9.Use Adversity To Further Your Own Goals, How Mike Tyson carved a path through the ills of a troubled childhood, Sean Kernan, medium.com, Dec 4, 2019, https://medium.com/publishous/a-champion-unbroken-use-the-secret-to-mike-tysons-success-to-further-your-own-goals-9158dec973be

10.Stadler G, Oettingen G, Gollwitzer PM. Intervention effects of information and self-regulation on eating fruits and vegetables over two years. *Health Psychol*. 2010;29(3):274-283. doi:10.1037/a0018644

11.https://woopmylife.org/en/science

12.https://en.wikipedia.org/wiki/Gabriele_Oettingen

13.https://en.wikipedia.org/wiki/Mind-wandering

14.Killingsworth MA, Gilbert DT. A wandering mind is an unhappy mind. *Science*. 2010;330(6006):932. doi:10.1126/science.1192439

15.Brewer JA, Worhunsky PD, Gray JR, Tang YY, Weber J, Kober H. Meditation experience is associated with differences in default mode network activity and connectivity. *Proc Natl Acad Sci U S A*. 2011;108(50):20254-20259. doi:10.1073/pnas.1112029108

16. 12 Science-Based Benefits of Meditation, by Matthew Thorpe, MD, PhD, Healthline, July 5, 2017 https://www.healthline.com/nutrition/12-benefits-of-meditation

17.Making Real Connections in the Age of Social Media, New platforms aim to alleviate loneliness and promote honest conversation. Lara Otte, Psy.D., Dec 18, 2019, Psychology Today https://www.psychologytoday.com/us/blog/the-human-connection/201912/making-real-connections-in-the-age-social-media

18.Epley N, Schroeder J. Mistakenly seeking solitude. *J Exp Psychol Gen*. 2014;143(5):1980-1999. doi:10.1037/a0037323

19.Boothby, E. J., Clark, M. S., & Bargh, J. A. (2014). Shared Experiences Are Amplified. *Psychological Science, 25*(12), 2209–2216. https://doi.org/10.1177/0956797614551162

20. Saint Louis University. "Man's Best Friend: Study Shows Lonely Seniors Prefer Playtime With Pooch Over Human Interaction." ScienceDaily. ScienceDaily, 9 January 2006. <www.sciencedaily.com/releases/2006/01/060108215831.htm>

21. Ditzen B, Schaer M, Gabriel B, Bodenmann G, Ehlert U, Heinrichs M. Intranasal oxytocin increases positive communication and reduces cortisol levels during couple conflict. *Biol Psychiatry*. 2009;65(9):728-731. doi:10.1016/j.biopsych.2008.10.011

22. Cohen S, Janicki-Deverts D, Turner RB, Doyle WJ. Does hugging provide stress-buffering social support? A study of susceptibility to upper respiratory infection and illness. *Psychol Sci.* 2015;26(2):135-147. doi:10.1177/0956797614559284

23. Gregory N. Bratman, Gretchen C. Daily, Benjamin J. Levy, James J. Gross, The benefits of nature experience: Improved affect and cognition, Landscape and Urban Planning, Volume 138, June 2015, Pages 41-50, https://doi.org/10.1016/j.landurbplan.2015.02.005

24.Gregory N. Bratman et al., Nature and mental health: An ecosystem service perspective, *Science Advances* 24 Jul 2019, Vol. 5, no. 7, eaax0903, DOI: 10.1126/sciadv.aax0903
https://advances.sciencemag.org/content/5/7/eaax0903

25. Your Guide to Healthy Sleep, NHLBI Health Information Center, September   2011
https://www.nhlbi.nih.gov/files/docs/public/sleep/healthysleepfs.pdf

26. Boosting Your Serotonin Activity, Alex Korb Ph.D, Nov 17, 2011, Psychology Today, https://www.psychologytoday.com/us/blog/prefrontal-nudity/201111/boosting-your-serotonin-activity

www.ingramcontent.com/pod-product-compliance
Lightning Source LLC
Chambersburg PA
CBHW061816250726
48657CB00001B/459